Mary Eva.. oung

Born in Romford, Essex, Mary is a staff development consultant, specializing in women's issues. In the early eighties the increased fear of violence against women, and the murder of Sally Shepherd inspired her to conceive and pioneer Safe Women's Transport, to help women living under curfew go out again at night.

A decade on, the suicide of a teenager because she was 'too fat', highlighted the extreme pressure on all females to be an 'ideal' size. Mary started Diet Breakers to help women challenge and recover from the tyranny of thinness. She lives in Oxfordshire with her husband and three cats. She has one daughter and one grandson.

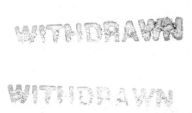

To the beauty and creativity of
all women and girls,
especially those of us who feel
we 'don't make the grade'.

In memory of my mother
Nellie Young and my
mother-in-law Clarissa
Blyth Evans.

Diet Breaking

Having It All Without Having To Diet

Mary Evans Young

Hodder & Stoughton

Copyright © Mary Evans Young 1995

The right of Mary Evans Young to be identified as the
Author of the Work has been asserted by her in accordance
with the Copyright, Designs and Patents Act 1988.

All cartoons © Viv Quillin

'I've got some growing to do' first published in
The Diet Free Diet Book by Janet Hunt, Green Print.

'One bite and I'll go straight to your hips' first published
by Cath Tate cards.

First published in Great Britain in 1995
by Hodder and Stoughton
A division of Hodder Headline PLC

10 9 8 7 6 5 4 3 2 1

A CIP catalogue record for this title is available
from the British Library.

ISBN 0 340 63790 0

Typeset by Hewer Text Composition Services, Edinburgh
Printed and bound in Great Britain by
Cox & Wyman Ltd, Reading, Berkshire

Hodder and Stoughton
A division of Hodder Headline PLC
338 Euston Road
London NW1 3BH

Contents

Acknowledgements

This book would not have been written without the help and support of Derek Evans. He has literally been with me every step of the way – from brainstorming the chapter breakdowns to editing my writing. He is my greatest ally, and his commitment and support to me, to Diet Breakers and to ending the tyranny of thinness have given me the strength and determination to keep going – especially when I felt I was banging my head against a wall or I was threatened by the diet industry.

When the publisher commissioned me to write this book I was given four months to do it. We had both had a very busy year, and had planned a five-week break. I could only write the book if I used my holiday time. Derek found a solution: we bought a lap-top computer, a mobile printer and a big bag, and we took the book on holiday with us. It is a measure of Derek's allegiance and his generosity that, instead of climbing mountains and playing in the sea and doing all the things he enjoys on holiday, he got up at six o'clock every morning to work along with me, reading, editing and checking my work.

There are a lot of people I want to thank. Firstly all the women who have taken part in my workshops and courses, from whom I have learnt and shared so much. The thousands of Diet Breakers supporters around the world who have endorsed my belief that change is possible. The hundreds of women who have written letters or completed questionnaires telling me their experiences. I have read them all, and only space prevents me from including everyone.

My daughter, Liza, provided me with an efficient press cutting service, and I appreciated her telling me I could do it and that she is proud of me. The love, support and enthusiasm of my dear friends Maud and Bill Cook – for me, for Diet Breakers and for this book – has been unswerving. Maud read through every letter and questionnaire to ensure I did not miss out any important areas. She was my sounding board and was not averse to telling me when I was becoming too strident. Bill kept the delicious fish pies and pasta coming and was my bridge partner when we needed a break from the book. My cousin, Derek Young, analysed the data from returned DB questionnaires and produced graphs and statistics.

I also want to thank the following people: Maggie Pearlstine 'for seeing it' when I first thought about writing a book, and for her loyalty and advice which has gone way beyond her role as literary agent; and nutrition researcher Jane Vigus, who checked my 'advice' in Chapters 3 and 5 and gave me her thoughtful comments generally. My friend and osteopath Bea Pike helped me with the section on stress, image consultant Penny Medley with the section on image, Stan Grant with the model of oppression, Sue Dibb and Tom Sanders with research, Diana Ross with research (particularly relating to government health policy), and Erika Smith with the section on massage as well as giving me lots of cuddles. Muriel Marcham provided efficient administrative back-up. Viv Quillin's understanding and feeling for the subject are reflected in her smashing cartoons. For their enthusiasm and ideas, thanks to Shelley Bovey, Beverley Bramwell, Sue Sharpe, Jo Ind, Rebecca Herisonne, Linda Taylor, Janet Goodall, Kate Greenway, Ros Juma, Jan Long, Di Smith, Gill West, Liz Sokoski, MaBel Dawson, Silvia Kogan, Gail Kavanagh, Frances Young, Joanna Strangwayes-Booth, Liz Sheppard, Sue Kerwan, Susan Martin, Dorothea Henwood, Tania Coombs and Linda Omichinski. I am also grateful to Sue Hyams and Mike Locke for their comments on my original draft chapter, to Heather Wetzel for her dedication and support in the early days of Diet Breakers, to Rowena Webb at Hodder & Stoughton for her encouragement and support, to Esther Jagger for her careful editing and to Dawn Bates for handling the last minute changes. Finally, thanks to Ray Marcham who looked after our three cats for five weeks whilst we were away writing it.

Foreword

We welcome this, the first book which genuinely deals with the diet scam – without being yet another diet book in disguise.

Great book! Full of tools and tips for those who still need convincing – fat or thin. Unlike many books this one will be read by the unconverted as well as by men and women – the tyranny of bodies affects us all and if we break out we can all experience life and beauty in its wide variations of form and richness of detail.

Much more fun.

This book is full of food for thought.

Dawn French and Helen Teague

Introduction

Despite considerable changes in their economic power in society over the last thirty-five years, women are still seen as objects. Intelligent, capable, successful, brave, hard-working women are judged primarily on their physical appearance. The result is that many women feel they have failed this intense public scrutiny and are ashamed of their bodies.

As I write, literally millions of women and girls will be counting calories, fighting the flab, pinching an inch, feeling the burn – or, if not, the consequences (ugly and unattractive). Of course, not all these women are unattractive and ugly, but they feel they are. The problem has reached epidemic proportions: women now hate themselves so much that they are constantly dieting and depriving themselves of healthy, enjoyable food, or punishing themselves through over-exercise, or being cut by a surgeon's knife – and boring themselves and everyone else to tears by their obsession with their weight.

For the last thirteen years I have worked as a management and staff development consultant. One of my areas of specialization is women's career development. I set up the organization called Diet Breakers because of a combination of factors: I had spent the best part of twenty-five years not liking my body, on and off diets before managing to break free, and I realized from listening to the women on my courses that most of them were suffering too.

I was called 'fatty' at school. I put up with the name-calling for quite a while, and then one day I lashed out – I hit a girl who was shouting out at me. Word of 'the fight' spread quickly through the school. Suddenly the name-calling stopped, and the reprieve from the onslaught was wonderful. I suspected they still had the same thoughts – but they were frightened of getting their ears boxed, and, anyway, the damage to my self-esteem and body image was already done. By the time I was twelve I felt very unhappy with my developing body.

When my mother took me to get my first bra I persuaded her to buy me a roll-on girdle too. I wriggled and struggled myself into the reinforced elastic tube with suspenders hanging from the bottom, and I felt great. Admiring myself as I stood in front of the mirror – all lumps and bumps had miraculously disappeared under the determined strength of the roll-on. I was tall and smooth from the waist down – because the flesh had been forced upwards and I now had the equivalent of a lower, second-level bust.

The roll-on should have been called the roll-up, because when I sat down all hell broke loose! Since at that age I didn't yet wear stockings to hold the garment down around my hips and buttocks, the wretched thing would roll up and up until it ended up a hot, tight elastic sausage roll around my waist. Not at all what I had intended. I was prepared to put up with the discomfort, but now I had the four-tier look: I had my breasts, the enlarged 'spare' tyre, the sausage roll and my belly. I was forever nipping into the toilets at school to pull it down. In desperation, I would even attempt to wriggle myself free under my desk. I put up with this for about six months before my mother relented and allowed me to wear stockings to school – a great expense since they laddered easily and we did not have much money. So I fixed the ladders with bright red nail polish and luxuriated in my new relative comfort.

From the age of about fourteen I started dieting. I lost a bit of weight, but by the time I was sixteen I was back to size 18 (American 16), where I stayed until I was twenty-one. Then one night I was watching *This Is Your Life* on television, and Eamonn Andrews was presenting the life of a famous jockey. One of the guests from his past life spoke from behind the curtain, and the jockey scratched his head as he racked his brain to find a name to fit the voice. What struck me was the man's brilliant suggestion for keeping the jockey's weight down: 'You can eat whatever you like so long as you don't swallow it . . . or put your fingers down your throat afterwards.'

'Wow!' I thought, 'That's fantastic! What a simple solution.' And, to augment my dieting, I took the trainer's advice and vomited two or three times a month for several years to assist me in my pursuit of weight loss.

I went from about 12 stone 8 pounds (176 pounds) in 1966 to 9 stone 8 pounds (134 pounds) in 1969. My weight then settled at around 10 stone 8 pounds (148 pounds). I was size 14 (American 12), and 5 foot 10 inches tall. Most people said I looked good. However, I still hankered to get down to size 12 – despite people telling me I did not look well when I was that thin. Apart from a couple of years in the mid-seventies, I maintained this weight level, mostly through restrained eating, for about fifteen years.

Throughout the seventies I belonged to a number of women's groups.

The discussions at our meetings were different from those of usual political meetings. We did a lot of consciousness raising – CR, we called it. We discussed our experience: what it meant to grow up female, what we wanted for ourselves and our daughters and society generally. We talked about politics and education and housing and wealth and health and art. We embraced the concept of taking responsibility for ourselves and our health. We talked about orgasms and sex and abortions and fashion and underwear and make-up and clothes and hairstyles and shaving our legs. We discussed Chinese foot-binding, the Hindu practice of suti or widow-burning, and female genital mutilation. One night we discussed for at least two hours the politics of blow drying our hair. Yet never once did we discuss dieting or size.

When Susie Orbach's book, *Fat Is a Feminist Issue*, came out I remember a number of people talking about it. One insightful woman said, 'Fat *is* a feminist issue – and not just the way Susie Orbach says.' And that was it.

Looking back now, it seems strange that I should sit through all these discussions and never bring up dieting, body image, size and weight as legitimate topics for discussion. I see it as a measure of the level of our oppression that I didn't – and neither did anybody else at the meetings I went to.

Regretably, that's where we are still at. We have yet to question, challenge and reject the concept that a full life for women is only achieved through an empty body. To me dieting is a form of western foot-binding. This is not to deny that foot-binding and genital mutilation are very important matters, but I wonder now whether we weren't focussing on the mistreatment of 'other' women's bodies as a diversion from dealing with our own hurt and mistreatment.

During the first half of the eighties I was still a 'restrained eater' on a low fat diet. I spent much of the decade developing my inner resources through workshops, assertiveness training, counselling groups and personal therapy, and I was in therapy training for six years.

In 1989 I spent a week at a health farm in Suffolk. It was a beautiful country house with elegant furniture, swimming pools and lovely gardens. The mornings were spent in our dressing gowns as we were moved swiftly through the beauty treatments: Turkish baths, steam baths, massage, water jets. The afternoons were a combination of relaxation and optional extras: leg waxing, facials, manicures, body toning and so on. In the evenings we were free to chat and walk in the grounds, or wander to the nearest pub. I spent from Sunday to

Wednesday fasting, drinking only lemon barley water, with a special treat of lemon and honey for tea. On Thursday I had some toast and on Friday I enjoyed a delicious low fat food. Saturday was weigh-in day, lunch and home. I had lost more than 7 pounds, which everyone agreed was a great success. My bill was £600. I came home feeling proud of myself for keeping to the regime and pleased with the weight loss. My husband churlishly pointed out that anyone who did not eat for a week would lose weight, but I ignored the remark . . . until I had been home three days and found I weighed exactly the same as when I went away. I decided that my next £600 would be spent on a proper holiday and resolved not to diet any more.

Over the last six years I have been learning to unravel the tangle of my emotional and physical hungers and to try to give myself what I want and need. I have been learning to accept and love my body, and I have been fighting the tyranny of thinness for the benefit of myself and all women.

'But what has happened to your size?' I am often asked. And I always answer: 'Why don't you ask what has happened to *me*? Because the size question is only relevant when we are in the diet mentality.'

I have been continuing to find myself. I have been learning to dance. I have been learning to feed myself and free myself from guilt. I have been learning to bite back and enjoy freedom. I have found my natural size, which is lower than when I was on and off diets and higher than when I was vomiting. More importantly than size is that my body feels more compact. For the first time in my life it feels right for me. I am my size.

This book is for women who want something different. It is for ordinary women of all sizes who feel unattractive or miserable, and who are constantly thinking of, talking about, and going on and off diets, or putting things off until they lose weight.

It is also for those women who are constantly comparing themselves to other women, and for the millions of women who have been on the receiving end of rude comments, have felt hurt and have had little or no support to deal with it. I hope, too, that women who are termed over-eaters, under-eaters, compulsive eaters or secret eaters, anorexic or bulimic, may also gain some support and useful guidance. My aim in writing this book has been to help motivate women to step off the roller coaster of diets and disasters, so that we can get on and enjoy our lives now.

1

The Tyranny of Thinness

You show me a woman who wants to be thin for her health and I'll show you a man who buys Playboy *to read the articles.*
Ellen Goodman, *Boston Globe*

'Thin is best' has become a powerful message in women's and girls' lives. I call it 'The Tyranny of Thinness' because its effect is to leave the majority of women and girls dissatisfied with their bodies. Negative thoughts and behaviour follow: we are forever wondering what others think of us, and whether we pass muster; and, most dangerously of all, we begin to develop unnatural eating patterns. The tyranny can dominate our lives if our thoughts are constantly about what we are eating and our weight. We can feel hurt at the merest negative comment about our looks, and crumple if we have failed to attain our God-given target weight. The pursuit of slenderness is draining, tiresome and a massive diversion from the real joys that life has to offer.

It caught me young. I think I was about nine or ten when I came home from school unhappy because some of the other children had called me 'fatty'. My mother sent me back with instructions to tell those kids, 'Sticks and stones may break my bones, but names will never hurt me.' So I swallowed my tears, put on a brave face and went back and shouted at them what my mother had said.

It was useful to have some ammunition to answer back with, but the message wasn't really true: their taunts hurt me like crazy. I knew already that to be 'fat' was bad. By that tender age I had absorbed the message that 'thin is best' and believed I didn't make the grade. I was hurt by the other children's comments, and so I hurt myself. I told myself I was ugly and unworthy. Now, when I look at photographs of myself taken then, I see a lovely ordinary little girl.

The tragedy is that it took me until I was well into my thirties to start healing the hurts and building my self-esteem and confidence, to start respecting and liking my body and to focus on positive aspects of myself. Increased self-respect has caused me to become increasingly irritated, for myself and other women, with the pressures we all have to endure to look and act a certain way: unhealthily thin and vulnerable. This letter from Cressida is typical of many that I receive at Diet Breakers. 'I have been dieting on and off for the past twenty-seven years, and would be grateful for any information that you can provide me with in order to stop this self-inflicted persecution which was imposed on me at a very early age, and which has led me into a trap that is now very difficult to get out of.'

No one escapes the threat of the tyranny. Ninety per cent of females diet at some stage in their lives. Whatever our size, most of us are caught. We have been conditioned to desire thinness at virtually any cost. Knowing you are not alone can be the first step in feeling better and fighting back.

Self-image, self-delusion

Advertisers tell us that aspirational images sell products. I ask, is it 'aspirational' for women and girls to be half-starved and obsessed with their bodies, their weight and what they had to eat last night? Those glitzy fashion photographs are a denial of reality. Behind the scenes we have social vomiting, women cutting their bodies to change their shape and girls damaging their healthy growth by dieting. For tabloid newspapers and women's magazines, slimming features are bog-standard staples. Attitudes are changing for the better, but many journalists of both sexes still need convincing that this is an issue for all women, regardless of size.

At Diet Breakers we receive numerous requests from the media for interviews with 'real women', to provide human interest stories. But journalists are often reluctant to interview average-sized or slim women because it doesn't suit their 'angle' – be it 'fat is beautiful' or 'shocking anorexics'. To portray dieting as solely a 'fat' issue denies the suffering of all those women who are trapped in the diet cycle and increases prejudice against fat women. Equally, pictures of women suffering with anorexia, however newsworthy, deny the trap that the majority of women find themselves in, and ignore the existence of links between dieting, eating disorders and fat oppression.

With the current anti-diet newsworthiness, an example of the media missing the mark and perpetuating the status quo was the story of Pam and John who were featured in a women's magazine. The headline of the article was: 'I love you just the way you are.' It was going to be, apparently, upbeat and inspiring, telling how Pam (size 18) and John fell in love and that he had never wanted her to lose weight. The interview was done and a photographer spent an evening taking shots of the couple. Each one was carefully set up and the photographer first took a Polaroid snap. Between the photographic session and publication of the article Pam showed me the half-dozen photographs of her and John. In two of them the couple looked really lovely: happy and smiling, obviously in love. But in some of the others John appeared to be pinned between the wall behind him and Pam in front of him. Guess which picture was published? Yes, that's right, one of John pinned against the wall. So the photograph gives the impression of the man being swamped by the woman.

The tyranny is so successful that most of us do not question it or rebel against it. Instead we knuckle down and accept it. We lay ourselves open to being hurt and abused by the merest comment because our identity, our self-esteem and our confidence are so closely connected to our appearance. A woman attending one of my management training courses said, 'The cruellest thing you can say to someone is, "You've put on weight".' When I asked her why, she replied, 'Well, nobody wants to be told they are getting fat, do they?' That woman had a point. Such is the tyranny that people who are told they are putting on weight often believe they are getting fat, even if it's not true.

A letter from Rachel said,

I am twenty-seven years old and have suffered in secret for the past eighteen months, ever since my 'friend' said that I looked fat. From that day on I have been on so many diets I've lost count. A year ago I was taken to my local doctor as I'd lost 1½ stone (21 pounds). My

doctor gave me a couple of boxes of Complan and sent me home.
Every time I eat I make myself sick. At other times I can go for days
without eating anything.

Because women and girls are not satisfied with their bodies,
many of them believe they are fat when they are not, including
those who are actually underweight. According to Naomi Wolf,
another of *The Beauty Myth*, a survey undertaken in 1985 con-
cluded that 90 per cent of respondents thought they weighed too
much. The negative feelings we have about our own and other
women's bodies are expressed obliquely in everyday comments
such as, 'You're looking really nice – have you lost weight?'
What am I meant to understand from that? That I only look
nice if I'm thinner, and woe betide me if I put any weight back
on? For a comment like 'You've got such a pretty face' read 'Any
attractiveness about your face is negated by your body.'

It's important to recognize these back-handed compliments for
what they are: a symptom of the tyranny that's wormed its way into
our psyche to the extent that we don't challenge it. We are used
to being ridiculed and insulted, sometimes biting our tongues and
mostly resigning ourselves to subtle and not so subtle abuse from
all directions.

From the historical viewpoint, the current obsession with thinness is whimsical. In the nineteenth century slim women were
pressured to appear *larger* than their natural size, and inflatable
rubber garments (complete with dimples) for the back, calves,
shoulders and hips were available. A hundred years ago the bustle
was a modish 'must have' to embellish the behinds of the less well
endowed.

Slimness first became fashionable in the early twentieth century,
although plumpness was still regarded as a sign of good health. In
the twenties women started binding their breasts to achieve the
flat-chested flapper look. The culture of slimming really took hold
after the Second World War, initially in the USA where the health
industry, taking its cue from insurance companies, urged the nation
to lose weight for its health.

Dieting promises success through slenderness. Yet in reality
most people find it impossible to maintain a weight lower than
their 'natural' weight. We feel ashamed of our bodies, and just
making the decision to go on a diet can be a quick and easy

way of alleviating that shame. Then, when the diet fails, we feel disappointed and ashamed again. It has become women's duty to diet and be thin – and the only thing stopping you from achieving it, you are brainwashed into believing, is you! Not to be thin, therefore, means failure.

Sharing feelings of guilt through failure and not being attractive enough becomes part of the diet ritual that keeps us hooked. One typical newspaper survey found that when women get together 70 per cent of their conversation is likely to revolve around dieting and slimming. We can, and do, talk about dieting just like the weather – to total strangers, safe in the knowledge that they will have something to say. It's even become a service to the community – we can raise money for charity by organizing or participating in a sponsored slim!

Talking about dieting can be reassuring, but it is a false sense of security because the nature of the tyranny is so competitive that it only works when you're failing. If you become one of the 4 in 100 successful dieters, you are out of the group. You no longer qualify for membership of the 'if only' club, and everyone else will envy you like crazy. In a familiar television commercial two women are amiably discussing the merits of low fat cheese spreads; in real life they would probably be secretly competing with each other over their size and weight.

Perhaps another reason why we talk about weight, dieting and thinness as much as we do is that it causes us a great deal of stress and angst. It's a cultural norm in which the suffering and negative effects are not acknowledged, and it is largely unknown to men.

The pursuit of thinness is more than just a matter of body size. It's about being acceptable, attractive and successful. The media confirm this for us with acres of column inches and hours of air time devoted to commenting upon women's clothes, appearance and weight.

In the glare of the media

When Lady Diana Spencer became engaged to Prince Charles she was described by the press and TV as an attractive and pretty young woman with a most becoming smile and a 'homely' disposition. She worked in a private kindergarten and as a nanny with an American

family, but we received no information about her skills or her work
because the media were more interested in her looks and what
she wore: a woman's appearance is how she'll be judged. First
there was the famous royal blue engagement suit, and then the
infamous photograph of her holding a child and wearing a long,
flowing, semi-transparent skirt. At this time Diana was probably
dress size 14 (American 12).

Almost overnight Diana transformed herself. Her hair became
blonder, she grew very image-conscious, and she lost weight. She
was congratulated on her new sophistication. She became a clothes
horse for the media, a vehicle for running commentary on her
appearance, attire and fashion statements. When the paparazzi
track her down working out in a gym or swimming, they report on
her body shape and her size. Even when she was pregnant there was
no let-up. The wife of an earlier Prince of Wales, Wallis Simpson,
once famously said: 'One can never be too rich or too thin.' Women
took on board the thin part of the statement, and the diet industry
made itself rich. Of course 'one' can be too thin. If we become too
thin we die. If we spend our lives trying to become too thin, the life
goes out of us. And so it was for Diana. Once, she lost too much
weight for the media. There was mock concern for her wellbeing
when it was suspected that she might be suffering from anorexia
or bulimia, and she was criticized for playing with her food and
for her faddish eating. Diana had gone too far – she had dieted
too much. She couldn't win. It was a pointed reminder to all of us
that our margin of acceptability is very narrow and non-negotiable,
and that failure invites a heavy penalty.

In contrast, Diana's sister-in-law Anne is reported in the press
for her work with charities such as the National Autistic Society
and Save The Children, and for her sporting activities – although
this was not always the case. She used to be vilified for her brattish,
Hooray Henrietta behaviour and her looks. Undoubtedly she has
worked at being taken seriously and it has paid off. The media now
report what she does, rather than what she looks like. We do not
know whether she is five pounds lighter today than yesterday, or
whether she was wearing tangerine or lime green. Anne is taken
seriously for who she is and what she does.

When Sarah Ferguson and Prince Andrew were courting I was
intrigued. Here was a woman who seemed to be breaking the
tyranny. From television pictures and photographs she looked an

average-sized woman. She was probably dress size 14–16 (American 12–14). I remember once seeing her wearing a gathered, calf-length skirt and a navy blue top with a large sailor collar. She had just finished a day's work at a publishing firm and was happily skipping along, smiling at the photographers and film crews. The world could see she was a woman in love. The reason she made such a strong impression on me, and why this image has stayed with me, is precisely because she looked so ordinary and so happy. She was a living contradiction of the 'thin' edict: she had escaped the tyranny. Here was proof that you don't have to be thin to marry your prince.

But, alas, my hopes and expectations soon turned to disappointment. The press started to pull Sarah Ferguson apart, remarking on her hairstyles, her size and shape, her style and dress sense. She seemed to reel under this bombardment, as most of us would. We saw first an astonishing array of ill-fitting clothes and then the grisly facts and pictures to go with them, as we witnessed her disappearance amongst an ever-increasing welter of exercise and weight-reducing regimes from Callanetics to hypnosis, swimming, gym and magical indoor pyramids.

Through the tabloid press I became a voyeur with the rest of the world as poor Sarah Ferguson changed into a very different (and thin) person. It is worth remembering that, although she initially achieved a waiflike figure, it was no insurance for a happy marriage. Many women believe they will be happier and life will be much brighter, if not exactly a bed of roses, if they could just lose weight. It simply is not true. Sarah has since regained much of the weight she lost and is again in the firing line. Meanwhile, Prince Andrew largely escapes vicious, negative and hurtful comments about *his* size.

Any woman in the public arena, be she a royal or a celebrity, is there to be sized up. Take Liz Taylor: pictures and articles chronicling her size and her relationship to food and dieting are commonplace. (A photograph of a 'fallen star' – which means 'fat' – fetches a premium price in the press.) We see her fat and in a wheelchair and we are encouraged to feel both sadness for her and a let-down for ourselves, because she is a star and we don't like to see her suffer. Or do we? 'She's rich and famous, and look at the state of her.' So long as she is thin, we will all want and love her . . . and aspire to be like her.

This message is not lost on ordinary women. Already feeling a bit insecure, we know we need to be loved. In a recent tabloid newspaper headline about television personality Amanda de Cadenet we were told she was 'looking "swell" [for "swell" read "fatter than usual"] . . . out on the town, seven weeks after the birth of her daughter Atlanta.' The message to readers was, 'Amanda has lost her original shape – will she get it back?' And by buying into Amanda's fatness we can feel a bit better about ourselves – either 'We're all in the same boat', or 'Thank goodness I'm not like her.' The critical treatment of the royals, Liz Taylor, Judy Finnigan, Amanda de Cadenet or Kathleen Turner when they put on weight serves to chastise and tyrannize the rest of us.

Oprah Winfrey has shared with the public her experiences, her successes and failures around food, weight and size. Oprah's show is shown in Britain twice a week, and every day in America. She is the highest-paid woman in television today. And in my book she deserves to be. She is sensitive, funny, in touch with real issues and real people. She is so popular that people queue to be in her audience, let alone to be a guest. She has her own production company based in Chicago, she is the boss.

These are impressive achievements for any woman anywhere. But Oprah Winfrey has dealt with many more obstacles in her life and career than the average media personality. For a start she's a woman, so she'll have had to deal with sexism. She's also black, so she'll have had to deal with racism. She came originally from the deep south of the USA and, as many Americans acknowledge, there is a distinct northern prejudice against southerners. She had many changes in her life as a child, moving between her parents and her grandparents. At the age of eight she was raped, and at fourteen she gave birth to a stillborn child. Somehow she managed to pull herself through and become a stunningly successful woman. Yet despite all this, Oprah said that her greatest achievement was losing weight.

If ever we needed an example of the way women are tyrannized into being thin, Oprah Winfrey is that example. In one fell swoop all those years of pain, hard work and achievement were swept away because she was not size 10.

Over the last couple of years Oprah regained the weight she lost, and now she has lost it again. This time she recruited the support of a personal trainer to help her exercise and train every day, and she eats 'delicious' low fat food prepared by Rosie, her personal cook. Articles in magazines and a book promote Rosie's menus – they worked for Oprah, they can work for you.

Oprah is a warm, caring and compassionate woman. In her efforts to help others she is falling into the trap of believing that thin is the only natural way to be. Oprah connected her body size and relationship to food to unresolved emotional issues, and this is true for many women – but not all. Unwittingly, Oprah is becoming part of the oppression. In her shows audiences clap and cheer her weight loss and that of others. Many of her shows focus on self-acceptance and self-esteem. I would like to see Oprah focus on the tyranny of thinness as a major hurdle in the path of self-acceptance.

The tyranny that destroys relationships

We have taken on board the message that 'Thin is good, fat is bad', and it distorts our views of ourselves and other women. On a bus one day I overheard a conversation between a mother and her daughter. The older woman was describing a recent discussion with her next-door neighbour about her marital problems. My heart sank as I heard the advice being given: 'I told her, "You've got to pull yourself together, lose a few pounds, get rid of your spare tyre." I mean, she can't blame him, can she, if he goes off with a more attractive woman when she starts putting on weight?' In other words, if a woman is carrying more weight than is regarded as acceptable, then she is a legitimate target for mistreatment by her husband and cannot rely on friendly support from her neighbour either. She is seen as deserving to be treated badly. Even worse, plenty of men are colluding and putting pressure on women too. The tyranny of thinness is a great equalizer. Women with very different experiences and from different walks of life can, and do, link up and talk about this issue. Which is what Christine and I did. A woman in her late thirties, she has been married to Brian for seventeen years, has two children and works for a building society, which she enjoys. I met her on a train journey to Newcastle when we sat opposite each other and struck up a conversation. I told her about my work, and she told me about her problem.

Her problem is in fact Brian, although she described it as a weight problem. She is an average-size woman, probably size 14 (American 12). She said she was size 12 when she got married and for a few years afterwards. Over the last thirteen years she had tried every conceivable diet, eating regime, milk shake and meal replacement to try to regain that size.

I suggested that her body might not want to lose weight – perhaps she's at her natural body size now. She immediately agreed with me and went on to explain, 'I'm fit and well, I like my food and don't really want to go on diets.'

'Why do you, then?' I asked.

'Because of my husband,' she replied. 'He just keeps on and on about me getting fat. I say to him, "Why don't you just accept me the way I am?" But then he says he does accept me – he just thinks I'd look better if I lost a bit of weight.'

I asked Christine if she had told Brian to back off.

'Yes,' she said in a weary voice, 'but he doesn't take any notice. He's always bringing home the latest diet book or cutting out articles about slimming and "Slimmer of the Year". So I go on another diet and then think, to hell with it, so I rebel and come off it. But I've got to do something soon as I don't want to go out with him these days because he is always looking at everything I eat. Even when we go to a restaurant with a group of friends, or go to a dinner party, if I eat a dessert I can feel his eyes burning into me from across the table. I don't look over, but I know he is looking. I can feel it. Then on the way home he'll start saying something like, "You didn't really need that apple pie." So I get angry and tell him to get lost, and then the whole evening has been ruined.'

I looked at her across the table in the train carriage, and tears were in her eyes as she looked down at her hands. 'I get angry with him because I feel he is always nagging at me and I want him to accept me for me, and I get angry and guilty at myself for not losing the weight.'

So is Brian using the tyranny of thinness as a weapon to hurt Christine? Or is Brian also a victim of the tyranny of thinness – does he need a partner who conforms to the current stereotypical beautiful image in order to feel OK about himself? I don't pretend to know the answer. Perhaps it's a bit of both. Clearly there are other things going on between them, and by focussing on the extra pounds their attention is diverted away from the real issue. Until one or the other of them faces that reality, I imagine that things will continue much the same as they have for the last thirteen years, with both of them thinking that Christine has a weight problem.

So it's not hard to accept that men like Brian are being influenced by the tyranny – if not directly, then indirectly, believing that an attractive female partner will enhance their position in some way. Many women feel insecure because of it, and understandably want to be more attractive than their male partners, even if the woman has a successful career herself. Women now have to be the best on all fronts: the best wife, the best lover, the best mother, the best worker, the best-looking. In other words, we have to do everything that men do and more besides – all on an empty stomach!

The changing status of women (and their hips)

Traditionally it has been relatively easy for men and women to measure their standing and success in society. For men status, income and possessions were the usual yardsticks. Women, on the other hand, did not have direct access to high personal income, so their beauty has been particularly useful as a means to access men's resources. And all around us Cinderella comes to life. Through the media we get the message that pretty women get the best men. If we just keep on dieting, then just like Cinders we too will get our own Prince Charming.

There seems to me little doubt that even a rich and powerful man's standing will shoot up when he steps out with an attractive woman, whether it's Richard Gere and Julia Roberts in the film *Pretty Woman*, or Carlo Ponti and Sophia Loren, or Aristotle and Jackie Onassis, or Woody Allen and Mia Farrow.

Fashion and beauty are so intertwined. For centuries, fashion has dictated women's body shapes with the help of bustles, corsets, girdles, brassieres, and now a revival of the Wonderbra. Women's bodies have to fit the fashion, rather than the other way round. We have been encouraged to be acceptable to others, but never entirely to ourselves. Twiggy's appearance on the fashion scene in the sixties is remembered as the beginning of the ultra-thin ideal body shape. A large part of her appeal lay in her childlike vulnerability. With her fair hair, enormous doe eyes, translucent skin and wafer-thin build, she would stand, pigeon-toed, her knees knocking. It was a very different look from the fifties' epitome of female attractiveness, Marilyn Monroe, although Marilyn projected vulnerability too with her fragile personality, tight skirts and high heels. With Twiggy, her personality didn't come into it. She didn't say anything. The message was conveyed through her appearance. In their different ways they were both very feminine and very dependent on strong men, and both had to work hard on their 'attractive' image.

Weight Watchers started in America in 1963 and was introduced to Britain in 1967. We have had thirty years in which to forget Marilyn Monroe, Jane Russell, Diana Dors and all the well-endowed 'ideal women' of the fifties. We have been busy watching, digesting, experiencing and developing new images and beliefs about what is regarded as attractive: Kate Moss would make Twiggy look positively well-nourished.

Something else was happening to women in the sixties, too. Ordinary women throughout the Western world were discovering a new kind of womanhood, a liberation of their bodies: freedom and independence through the birth control pill.

The Pill transformed women's lives. In thirty years we have seen massive changes in women's position in society. We are now living in a time of relative plenty, of sexual liberation and (relative) female emancipation, and a certain prestige is accrued from being thin. Thinness is a metaphor for resisting the excesses of consumerism: it projects an image of self-control, self-restriction and sexual androgyny. Unlike the tenets of consumerism, less is always best, and the stripped down, lean, dynamic woman is apparently primed to get her piece of the action.

Abstinence is seen as a virtue. In the fifties women were either 'good' or 'bad' depending on whether they were virgins, mothers or whores. They were expected to abstain from sex before marriage. Thinness has, to an extent, replaced virginity as the desirable female quality. Now, we are expected to abstain from food.

I believe the degree to which women have 'progressed' is illusory. The incredible success achieved in normalizing the values of slenderness and fatphobia tells me we haven't got very far at all. Sexual liberation has made it acceptable for us to be fed a daily diet of female images that thirty years ago would have been considered pornographic. Dieting is an attempt to change our bodies from the inside, so that we can present the naturally ideal body shape. Women now show more flesh and don't wear girdles (which shaped our bodies from the outside), and therefore give others a fairly accurate impression of the female form underneath the clothes. This exposure, warts and all, is then compared to the idealized, 'pornographic' images of women. Not surprisingly, most of us don't come up to scratch. We have bellies and thighs, though you wouldn't think so from some current television commercials – boyish hips and a flat, almost caved-in stomach reinforce the message. In an age of plenty, with the accompanying moral fear of sloth and weakness, the strong-willed and able can apparently, like modern technology, overcome any imperfections and succeed.

In the sixties, when the women's movement was making ground, we started wearing practical clothes: flat shoes – great for getting around safely and quickly (we could actually run), as well as good for our backs. We wore long skirts, jeans or dungarees, which were perfect for everyday women's tasks such as doing the shopping and taking the kids to the park. But this fashion was soon denigrated as the women's libbers' and lesbian look. We were encouraged to despise it, and were told that the women who wore it were ugly and unfeminine.

Looking back, I can see how I was attracted to the idea that there was nothing stopping us becoming more successful, in the sense that we could be fit, strong and healthy and get 'proper' jobs like men do. What I realize now is that we have constructed the appearance of health and energy and hidden what lies beneath: the stress, anguish, pain and health risks of trying to achieve it. We struggle to counter the daily semi-sexual images of women so that we can be judged on our achievements. At work we wear jackets and shoulder pads that disguise our natural female shape so as to fulfil one of our other roles, that of career woman. Flesh is feminine, but flesh is also now seen as 'fat', which is weak and soft. As a consequence, one of the main attributes that distinguish us from men has, for the 90 per cent of us who still have body flesh, become very negative, and subsequently guarantees us second place in the pecking order.

The recession of the late eighties brought with it rising unemployment and the waif look. Dr Roberta Seid, a lecturer on the Program for the Study of Women and Men in Society at the University of Southern California, says, 'We are encouraged to adopt the behaviour and attitudes of the anorexic – it's only a question of degree.' The waif's body is saying, 'I am no threat. I'm harmless, vulnerable, pliable.' To make the point she is frequently seen on her knees or up against the wall advertising products such as perfume or clothing. In *The Beauty Myth* Naomi Wolf says, 'A cultural fixation on female thinness is not an obsession about female beauty but an obsession about female obedience . . . and about how much social freedom women are going to get away with or concede.' Not eating enough immobilizes us. Striving for an impossible ideal diverts us. And constantly comparing ourselves with other women divides us.

Who pays the piper? I think it is extraordinary that we women should starve, cut or attempt to alter our bodies for fashion. Haven't we got things a bit cock-eyed? Whatever happened to the edict that he (or in this case she) who pays the piper calls the tune? I heard one fashion designer say he couldn't design clothes for women over size 12. I would like to tell that designer: 'Learn, or else get another job!' Just imagine that you wanted a new pair of curtains and an interior designer said to you, 'Sorry, madam, I don't make curtains for your shape of windows. You'll have to get the builders in and have your windows remodelled.' You would probably think, quite rightly, that he or she was raving mad. Undoubtedly you would say, 'Get lost.' Yet, this in effect is what fashion designers are telling women. At the risk of sounding homophobic, which I am not, I wonder why so many of the gay fashion designers don't concentrate on designing clothes for men and youths – rather than designing clothes for women that make them look like twelve-year-old boys.

We have redefined what is and isn't fat. In haute couture you can buy clothes that are size 6 (American 4). Size 6 means hips that measure just 30 inches in Britain, 32 in America. The labelling and redistribution of garment sizes now suggest that sizes 6 and 8 are small, sizes 10 and 12 are medium, and size 14 is large. Size 16+ is outsize, and requires special shops and departments. This is despite the fact that 47 per cent of British women are size 16 or over. In other words, almost half the female population are being told they are abnormal and overweight. These aren't nice messages to receive, and are purely subjective. I say, 'Overweight for what and for whom?'

If we let it, our weight can become a thermometer to gauge how we feel about ourselves today and every day, because thinness has become the model for the successful modern woman. Dieting provides us with a challenge. Since only 4 in 100 can win the thin game, winning has become highly prized. Fashion clothing like the mini or the micro, with tank tops and skinny-ribs – the tighter the better – is victory dress for the wearer with nothing so nasty as excess flesh to hide. It reinforces our need to find the next magic weight loss solution. The rest of us must hunt the high streets for something a little less demanding, a little less revealing. Gone are the days when we were told, 'If you've got it, flaunt it.' Now, the message is, 'If you've got it (that is, any amount of "excess flesh") get rid of it – through dieting, vomiting, over-exercise or surgery if necessary. And if all else fails, hide it.' 'Excess flesh?' We are talking about women's bodies, not an extra pound of bacon that's fallen into the shopping trolley this week! The effect of all this is that women hide themselves away under their clothes and in the way they walk and move – or simply by not going out.

Against this backdrop, perhaps it is unsurprising that trendy nightclubs like Stringfellows are not over-welcoming to fat women. The 'sparkling' Mr Peter Stringfellow's ban was widely reported in the press. He saw a fat woman in his club one evening and asked one of his bouncers whether she was 'the loo attendant'. She was fat and was wearing what in his opinion were unattractive clothes and – wait for it – flat shoes. When I asked Mr Stringfellow himself on a radio programme what he had to offer women, he said he was 'fifty-odd, not bad-looking and [had] a ponytail.'

The health smokescreen

The obsession with thinness breeds rude and unkind remarks about fat people who are used by the diet industry as the fear factor: if you weaken you will end up like them. Fat people are there to be pitied and abhorred; we dislike our own bodies so much that we need someone – doesn't matter if we know them or not, because anyone will do – to look down on. Temporarily, at least, we can feel better about ourselves. We mask our dislike of fat with an expression of concern about the person's health.

I came across this smokescreen a couple of years ago when, just after the first International No Diet Day, I was invited to take part in a live television discussion with Professor Arnold Bender from Weight Watchers. When I arrived at the studio I found that the other guest was 'the-lady-always-wears-pink' journalist and dedicated dieter, Nina Myskow. Before the programme the presenter, the formerly New York-based Bob Friend, chatted to me in the green room about the show and put me at my ease.

It was the first sunny day of the year and the item started with footage of some fat people in America at a social gathering with their partners. Bob's opening question to me was, 'It's a hot day in London to be fat, isn't it?' I made the point that it was hot regardless of our size, and that most people who are dieting are not fat. Back came Bob with a remark about whether those people in the film were attractive or not. In one clean sweep all those people and their partners had been condemned for their size. Don't get me wrong – from this limited experience of Bob Friend I'd say he is a well-intentioned man. He tried to be fair during the debate and of course wanted a lively discussion for his show, but the effect of such a judgement can be devastating for anybody who because of their size is not feeling good about themselves. The chances are that they are leading restricted lives in order to avoid just such cruel and hurtful comments.

Nina Myskow, on the other hand, is a different kettle of fish. She said she was 5 foot 3 inches tall and that at one time she had weighed 175 pounds. She advocates dieting because she 'succeeded'. Nina stands out by being controversial and sometimes rude about people. On this programme she said that the people in the film looked like whales and were full of blubber. When I asked her why she was being so rude and unkind, back came that old chestnut of a reply: 'Well, it can't possibly be healthy.' In other words, anyone above UK size 12 (American 10) should be grateful, for the tyrants have only your best health interests at heart. There's nothing more boring than a born-again sinner (slimmer).

Let us here and now challenge the myth that if we don't diet we become overweight or obese. In some senses it achieves exactly the opposite effect. For instance, dieting causes us to become fixated with food. It also slows down our metabolism. Depriving ourselves of food can cause us to react by bingeing. And stopping dieting does not automatically cause weight gain.

Let us also challenge the myth about the health risks of being so-called 'overweight'. Researchers now believe that these dangers have been exaggerated. Being plump may even be a protection against some diseases, whereas weight fluctuation (yo-yoing) through dieting may lead to heart disease and even death. If you are heavy but fit you won't necessarily run any more health risks than thinner people. (See Chapter 3 for more on this important subject.)

The *real* health risk

Making rude comments about fat women feeds into the insecurities of all women. Since most women who are dieting are already thin they are obviously doing so for some other reason, and remarks such as 'Fat people are unattractive' only fuels their insecurities. 'Thank God I don't look like that,' you hear women saying. 'I couldn't stand him to talk about me like that,' or 'If I was size 18 I would commit suicide.'

Some people do commit suicide. I started Diet Breakers partly in response to reading about a sixteen-year-old girl who committed suicide because she could not face life being fat. That girl was size 14 (American 12). And in 1994 the media were full of the story of Michaela and Samantha Kendall, the twins who developed anorexia; Michaela lost her life to the disease. They said they had started dieting as young teenagers after being called fat. I have seen photographs of them at that time, and they were not fat.

I understand how these comments and thoughts come about. Oppressed people frequently internalize their own oppression (more on this in Chapter 6). If we are told something long enough and often enough, we eventually begin to believe it. Nina Myskow will almost certainly have internalized some of her weight and size oppression. It can, in the short term, help us feel better if we put someone else down.

I am not suggesting that every dieter ends up with an eating disorder, but every person with an eating disorder started out as a dieter. A common feature for women who are not dieting is to feel guilty after they have eaten. We eat the food and then we hate ourselves. We feel ashamed of our entire bodies, or of particular parts of them. Then we hate our entire selves because we were not strong enough to refuse the food in the first place, and we are ashamed that we have these feelings about something so apparently small and easy.

Let's kick the habit!

Undoubtedly women have achieved a lot in the last thirty years. We are getting more and better jobs, we are buying houses, we are no longer required to get our husband's permission to have a hysterectomy, we have a few more female politicians and there are more women in the public eye. Yet to an extent pleasure and pride in our achievements are whipped from under us when our main aim in life is to lose weight; and the means of achieving that success can often appear distorted in our own and other people's eyes.

The little voice box you can buy to go in your fridge reminds you, 'If you're thin, you'll win.' It also encourages us to believe its hard-hitting corollary – that our weight is responsible for our failures and disappointments. If you have one of those little voice boxes, here's what you should do with it:

1. Place one large sheet of newspaper on floor
2. Put voice box in centre of paper
3. Look at voice box from all directions
4. Take three deep breaths
5. Raise right foot
6. Bring right foot down heavily on to box
7. Twist and grind foot until plastic is nicely shredded ·
8. Stand back and admire your work
9. Wrap plastic in newspaper
10. Place bundle in bin

Bye-bye guilt, hello powerfulness, hello happiness, I think I'm gonna smile.

I believe that many women who are trying to be slimmer are not dieting because they are vain or because they really believe they will be more attractive or that their lives will be better as a result. I believe that many women who spend years on and off diets, with their weight going up and down, are desperate to escape the tyranny of thinness. That tyranny has become so much a part of our everyday lives that women stop eating and enjoying good food and instead feed themselves a diet of self-hatred – hating their bodies and draining their spirits.

Many of the things I describe as part of the tyranny of thinness may seem trivial individually. Yet nothing is in isolation. No comment or look ever stands alone. These individual, trivial things begin to mount up, limiting us, trapping us and punishing us by draining our confidence, self-esteem and energy. Regardless of whether we lose weight or not, any woman who is tyrannized becomes a shadow of her real self.

I've got news for the fashion industry, the media, the advertising industry, the diet industry, the food manufacturers, the potion peddlers, the pill pushers and the manic exercise gurus: women around the world have had enough. We are no longer prepared to accept your lies and negative messages. We are not ugly and unattractive. Walk down any high street next Saturday afternoon and see the variety and diversity of women's beauty.

I've got news for women, too: we don't need to diet to be healthy or attractive. We don't need to criticize each other or be tyrannized any longer. Save your money – don't waste it on ridiculous diets, regimes and lies, don't get sucked into the diet mentality. Get on with your life – right now. You deserve better, and you can have better – right now.

The tyranny of thinness has had its day.

2

The Hidden Evidence: Women's Dieting Experiences

Trapped for life

Hundreds of women have written to tell me their dieting histories. I have cried as I have read some stories, while others have made me feel outraged. I want people to know what women are going through. Our experiences need to be out in the open, not denied or hidden away, because they shed a completely different light on those dieting myths and illusions that we are so familiar with:

- It's natural and good for us
- It works
- It brings us happiness and success
- It boosts our confidence
- It stops us becoming obese

The youngest person to write to me was fifteen and the oldest seventy-nine. When I read the latter story I threw the letter down screaming, 'For heaven's sake, are we not free at any age?'

Many mothers have written about their daughters. One woman said her seven-year-old daughter asked if she could diet, and another said she was put on her first diet at six months and has been dieting ever since. Many women say they 'picked up the habit' at school, from their mothers or from magazines.

A number of men have written saying they have watched their wives or partners dieting, but have not known how to help them stop. A man from Birmingham wrote,

I wholeheartedly agree with your statement that slimmers do regain their weight and possibly much more. My wife has made her life a misery in trying to reduce weight; I have gone along with her wishes. However, as we are both in our late sixties I think it better to depart this life overweight and happy rather than miserable and trying to achieve the unattainable.

Over a period of two and a half years Diet Breakers sent out questionnaires to everyone who sent us a stamped addressed envelope. The questionnaire is at the end of this chapter, and you may like to complete it yourself. The statistics in this book are taken from 516 returned questionnaires.

The stories and experiences of the women and girls who completed the questionnaires, coupled with the thousands of letters we receive, has helped us gain a unique picture of the extent of dieting and the problems it's causing.

It is not an exaggeration to say that dieting is an epidemic, and most dieters are veterans of many failed weight loss regimes. Diets:

- wreck lives
- don't lead to permanent weight loss
- don't improve health
- are addictive
- can lead to serious eating disorders
- cause obsession with food, body and weight
- sap women's confidence, self-esteem and energy
- divert women from facing their real issues
- prevent them from fulfilling their potential
- affect all women and girls
- cost a fortune

Here is the evidence. This cross-section of case histories demonstrates the reality facing all women and girls in Western society today. I have resisted the temptation to use only 'dramatic' stories, as I do not want to sensationalize the problem by focusing only on extremes. Some of the stories are of course dramatic and very moving, while others are alarming because of their ordinariness. I believe most women will be able to identify with at least one of these case histories.

All bar two of those who supplied the relevant details are at

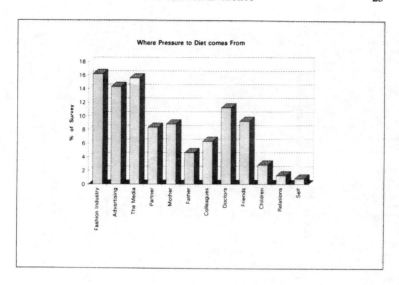

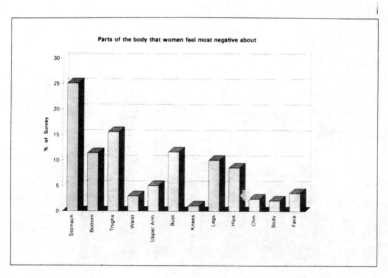

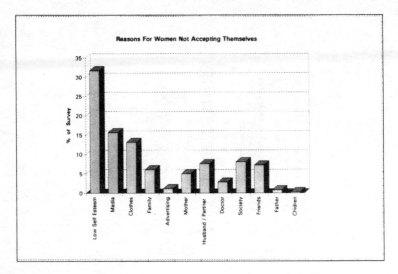

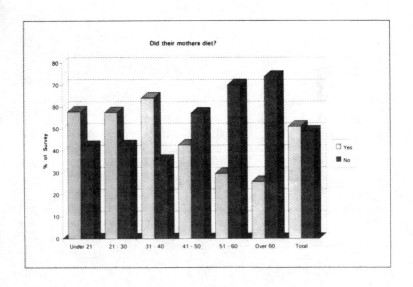

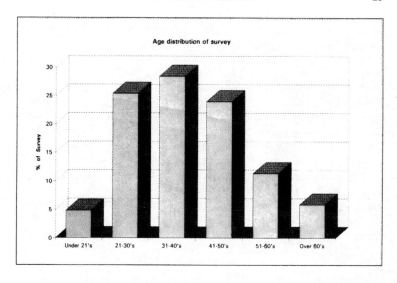

The graphs clearly show that the pressure to diet comes from the fashion, advertising and media industries.

what experts regard as a healthy weight for their height, yet they have still been unhappy with their body weight and shape and have therefore dieted. I do not accept that height and weight charts are an automatic guide to whether a person is healthy (more of this in Chapter 3). But heights and weights are given here with each woman's story, if they were provided in her response to our questionnaire, as I want to explode the myths that surround slimming.

These first four stories of Sue, Louise and Viv and Anne are typical of ordinary women leading ordinary lives who then get trapped in the diet cycle with no easy way out.

Louise

Height 5 foot 3 inches Weight 7 stone 12 lb–8 stone 3lb (110–115 pounds) Age Twenty-five Occupation Teacher

Three years ago I was about 10 stone and a good size 14, so I really should be happy with the size and weight I am – it usually depends on how my frame of mind is at the time. I never intentionally started to diet – I went to university and slowly it came off. I am now at the stage where I've been working in my first job for quite a while, and how I am about my weight has suddenly become a lot worse.

Right now I'm labelled as 'petite' and 'cute' – not me at all, really. I'm the typical blue-eyed, fair haired, okay-looking girl who should be more than happy with her appearance, but I just can't be. I'm always on the bathroom scales pondering how I can maybe lose a couple of pounds, and basically it's driving me crackers! I'm at the stage where I really do not know if I'm anorexic, bulimic, or just obsessed with dieting in general. I've tried to sit and analyse exactly why it could be a problem, but I don't seem to have got anywhere at all. I've tried to conquer all this by myself – you know, the food diaries, things I need to improve, etc. – but it just hasn't worked. The only good thing so far is that nobody has noticed the fact that I never really eat much – although my husband nudges me to eat things sometimes. I know that I am only harming myself and that being twenty-five years old and a teacher as well I should really be able to handle all this, but I'm a little worried that it'll turn into something bigger.'

Louise has seen the ad, tried the products and she's thin. The ads say she 'should' be happy now – but she isn't, and feels guilty.

Sue

Height Not supplied Weight Not supplied Age Not supplied Occupation Not supplied

I feel that I am in the 'diet trap'. I weigh myself at least three times a day and I constantly think about food, what I allow myself and what is 'forbidden'. All I want to lose is 5 pounds but I feel enormous and as if it's lots to lose. I've always had a weight problem, I'm always slimming, and I feel guilty if I eat anything 'naughty'.

About six years ago I joined Weight Watchers and lost 16 pounds in seven weeks. I felt wonderful – much more confident, and good in everything I wore. I kept the weight off for twelve months, though I was totally obsessed by it and it was an effort. I gained about 5 pounds and managed to control my weight – easier this time – and even though I gained 3 stone (42 pounds) whilst pregnant I lost it fairly easily. But I got a bit obsessed when I was only 3 pounds heavier than previously.

Since Christmas, when I gained 5 pounds, I have become totally obsessed about losing this weight. I'm so depressed because of it, and feel 'fat and fed up'. I think about food all the time, and look at other people to see how fat they are. I've bought an exercise bike to help, but despite daily use it's made no difference.

My boyfriend tells me I'm fine the way I am – I'm actually about the same as when we met or a little lighter. He can't understand my compulsion with my weight as he's never had to diet, ever, and eats 'naughty' things and gets away with it.

I really would like to join Weight Watchers again, but it's quite expensive and it may not really help me. I think that I really do need help now, because it is getting worse instead of better.

Sue's weight is the same as when she first met her boyfriend, or thereabouts. She doesn't say how old she is, but we do weigh more as we get older and it's perfectly healthy. In the diet mentality we have strict notions of 'good' and 'bad' food and find ourselves constantly comparing ourselves with other women.

Viv

Height Not supplied Weight 8 stone 7 lb (119 lb) Age Not supplied Occupation Not supplied

I am now the biggest I have ever been. I am trying hard not to succumb to a lot of negative thoughts I have about my body which leave me crying myself to sleep some nights (on a bad day). So I am finding it very, very difficult to feel good and stay at this weight.

We don't know her height, but if she's 4 foot 10 inches or over she's at a healthy weight. She is not alone in crying herself to sleep at nights.

Anne

Height 5 foot 5 inches Weight 8 stone 3 lb (115 lb) Age Thirty-one Occupation Not supplied

For the past nine years I have been constantly on and off diets. They say that as you get older the problem may disappear, but in my case it seems to be getting worse. At my weight I feel miserable and still feel that I could lose a few more pounds, even though everyone tells me I should put some on. Diet and exercise have become the priority in my life – everything else is worked around them. I have one meal a day in the evenings, with an apple for lunch, and that will be all I eat for the day. I do aerobics four or five times a week to burn up my calories and to increase my metabolism. I often binge when it gets too much and then take laxatives to rid my system of all the excess.

I have a loving husband who is at his wits' end and claims that I put my weight before everything else, including himself and our children. I don't drink any more and am very reluctant to go out for meals in case I over-eat. This is ruining my social life.

My friends are sick of hearing about my diets and how much weight I've lost. My family are worried and people at work have noticed a change in my behaviour.

Although I realize I have a problem, I cannot get rid of it overnight and it will take a long time. I want to change and go back to leading a normal life without having to worry what I eat all the time.

Another aspect of the diet mentality is obsessive exercise, in the false belief that this is healthy and will reduce weight. The rest of her life is on 'hold' and her relationships are suffering.

Allison

Height 5 foot 7 inches Weight Not supplied Age Sixteen Occupation Schoolgirl

I have always been a naturally slim person and at 5 foot 7 inches I had a figure that was the envy of many. It all began in November 1992 when a lot of my friends suddenly became concerned with their figures and began dieting in a big way. Of course with all the talk of food, body weight and shape I often got comments such as 'Oh, I wish I was so thin' and 'You're really lucky, you can eat what you want and yet you're so skinny.' It was true – I enjoyed food and could eat anything in huge quantities, and I wouldn't look or feel any different. We all sat in one big group at school lunchtimes tucking away. Then suddenly the trend changed to low calorie health food whilst I was still munching my white bread ham sandwiches saturated with margarine, with crisps and chocolate afterwards.

I studied home economics for two years and soon became very

conscious of my unhealthy eating habits. At every home economics lesson healthy eating was the central theme and my knowledge quickly became an obsession. I suddenly felt very pressurized into preserving my figure because so many people were envious of me. I was scared that they would lose lots of weight whilst I carried on naturally putting a little weight on because I was still growing. It also coincided with my older sister, who is naturally very plump, moving back home. She and my mum had always said, since I was a kid, that as soon as I became a teenager I would put weight on and fill out just like my sister did. It was a fact I'd had drummed into me, and now I became all too aware of it.

My sister was unhappy with her life, which made her very conscious of her figure and she carefully watched what she ate. From the very day she moved in I could see that she was jealous of my figure – even my mum agreed that it wasn't in my imagination. I may be wrong, but she was always unnaturally interested in what I ate and how much, and would only allow herself a treat to eat if I was having something too. This put me under more pressure because I wanted to show her how healthy my diet was, and every day it made me more aware of exactly what I was eating.

It could also have been caused by fear of growing up (which I am aware of) and exam pressure. Now my sister has left home again and I have new friends who enjoy their food and couldn't care less about their weight. Yet still I torture my mind about food, day in and day out.

Last January I was extremely underweight and my health was suffering. Since then I have put on over a stone and am now only a little underweight, yet mentally my problem is as bad as it was then. I've seen my doctor about it, but she seemed to patronize me. When she found out that I wasn't bulimic she gave me the impression that it was a trivial thing. I often talk to my mum about it, but it is hard for her to understand what goes through my head and I try not to worry her too much.

Lately I have started bingeing. I try to stop it, and my mum helps too, but I feel like I am beginning to lose control. I now live for food, when I wake up I plan all the nice food I can eat and I'm not content until I've eaten it. I feel as though I can get through the day if I allow myself to eat what I want. I only look forward to going out if good food is involved. I know that I can't go on like this both mentally and physically but I have run out of ways to stop myself pigging out, all my efforts seem to fail.

Allison, as a 'vulnerable' young woman likely to be concerned about her looks and weight, and with pressures in her school and home life is a prime target for the diet industry. Her story exposes the myth that dieting is done in the pursuit of healthy weight loss. She wanted to maintain/lose weight, terrified that she would lose her status and attractiveness if she put it on. It also highlights how well-intentioned nutritional information given at school can backfire. Instead of enabling young people to make healthy eating choices it can be used to justify obsessive eating – the vicious diet cycle, swinging from deprivation to bingeing.

Katy

Height 5 foot 8 inches Weight 10 stone 7 pounds–11 stone (140–154 lb) Age Forty-five Occupation Not supplied

I am trying desperately hard to *stop* thinking about food – I hate my body and food is an enemy. I wish, on a regular basis, that I didn't like food, that I didn't love the flavour and texture of food, that I hated all sweet things. I am trying to stop imagining that if I were thin everything would be all right, that I would suddenly love my body and that the self-revulsion would cease. I don't think anyone in my personal life has stopped me from accepting myself as I am, but I think magazines and advertising have done a great deal to help me form the opinion that my body is ugly and that anyone who finds it attractive must be perverse.

I am coming to terms with my obsession with weight, but what I am left with is anger – anger that the few precious years between childhood and true adulthood (fifteen to thirty) were robbed from me. I did have fun, of course, but so much time was lost and so many things were not done because I felt too fat to do them (the old theme – when I'm thin I'll reward myself by doing so-and-so).

Deborah

Height 5 foot 6 inches Weight 9 stone 10 lb (136 lb) Age Thirty-nine Occupation Not supplied

I have had difficulty in accepting myself as I am because I felt that, if I was thinner, then I would feel more attractive within myself and to other people.

My history with food is anything but brief, but in a nutshell it has completely dominated my life. I comfort eat (or did), and I would control what I ate to such an extent that I deliberately avoided going out for meals, using every excuse I could, as I was terrified of putting on weight.

I would wake up in the morning and think about food, and I would go to bed at night still thinking about food. I would starve/binge, and eat food in secret. Binges would start either because I was starving, or I would eat for comfort rather than deal with my problems.

My relationship with food was a love/hate one – I love food, but I hated what it did to my body (not any more, though). In May 1990, at 9 stone 2 pounds (129 pounds), I decided to go on a diet, as I wanted to weigh 8 stone 7 pounds (119 pounds). But this diet was different as well as low calorie – it was low fat.

I started to become obsessed with all aspects of my eating, and kept a book in which I recorded everything I ate, with the relevant calories and grams of fat, carbohydrates (of which I noted the amount that was sugar), protein and fibre. At the end of each day I would add up all the calories. I would then calculate the percentage of fat in my daily diet.

I repeated this analysis for carbohydrates, protein and fibre, to ensure I was eating 'heathily'! I did this every day for almost four months.

In January 1992 I weighed 7 stone 11 pounds (109 pounds). I still felt fat. Luckily my body decided to fight back, and I could no longer stick to this diet. I began to binge, and from June 1992 to April 1993 I entered the diet/binge cycle. In May 1993 I weighed 10 stone 9 pounds (149 pounds) and, as I said earlier, when I started the above diet I was 9 stone 2 pounds (128 pounds). So do diets lead to long-term weight loss? Do diets make you feel like a different person? Do they bring you happiness and a sense of wellbeing? *No, they do not*!

In answer to your question about whether my mother dieted – is the Pope Catholic? My mother must be a major shareholder in Weight Watchers by now.

Katy and Deborah are (or were) in a state of daily torture with their love/hate relationship with food. Katy expressed a virulent hatred of her body. Many adverts for diet products exploit this turmoil and the feelings of guilt and self-loathing.

Joan

Height 5 foot 8 inches Weight 10 stone 7 lb (147 lb) Age Fifty-four
Occupation Not supplied

My problems with food and dieting started at a very early age. When
I was eleven, and still at primary school, the school nurse decided I
needed some help as I was 'overweight'. My parents were contacted
and I was referred to a dietitian at the hospital. My mother dutifully
took me to see Mrs Finch, a very thin, hungry-looking woman of
about sixty-five.

Yes, I was too heavy and needed to lose weight, was her message.
My mother was issued with a diet sheet and given various instructions.
Every week we were to attend and I was to be weighed.

Mrs Finch frightened my mother somewhat, and that fear was
channelled into what I could and could not eat. My mother controlled
my food intake very carefully indeed, so that the necessary weight
loss would be recorded on the next visit to the clinic. Other children
were enjoying the odd sweet and piece of cake but for me they were
forbidden, so I have felt guilty about 'fattening' food ever since.

The weight I lost under Mrs Finch I quickly put back on, and when
I was sixteen another school nurse encouraged me to diet. Believe
me, I was never grossly overweight, but at impressionable stages in
my development a rather disturbing message was being sent to me:
'You must lose weight or else you won't get on very well.'

People advising me and 'encouraging' me to lose weight at such a
young age has screwed me up. I have been on diets constantly over the
last thirty years, as I find it difficult to accept that I am not overweight
and that for me there is nothing disgraceful about being a size 14.

At last I feel I am beginning to get to grips with myself. I have a
daughter of nine and I don't want her to end up like me – diet-crazy.
So I have stopped being obsessed by what I eat. My main topic of
conversation is no longer what I weigh or what I ate for dinner
last night!

So whose 'problem' was it really? Joan's mum's, Mrs Finch's, other
people's? In the end it turned into Joan's, and has lasted for over
forty years. Joan did not learn new behaviour or eating patterns,
if indeed she needed to, through Mrs Finch's chastisements. From
the age of eleven Joan has been encouraged to view her health
solely from a visual (size) perspective, rather than in terms of how
she was feeling.

Linda

Height 5 foot 2 inches Weight 14 stone 7 lb (203 lb) Age Thirty-six
Occupation Not supplied

I never really thought of a particular weight – it was a particular size I
fantasized about. I wanted a flat chest. My large bust has always been
a 'problem'. I've worn a bra since I was nine, so you can imagine what
PE, swimming and walking along the street could be like. For years I
yearned to have a bust measurement of around 32 inches and not to
need a bra.

When I was twelve I went on my first very low calorie diet. I was
prompted by a calorie sheet issued free by *Jackie* magazine and
an article it carried on dieting – the usual thing about 'shedding
those surplus pounds so you too can wear jeans and a T-shirt this
summer'!

I drew up my own 800 calorie-a-day diet sheet, and I was on the
diet for about five months. I am appalled that my mother let me do
it. I was only eleven, for goodness sake! I was still growing! That was
the beginning of the diet/binge syndrome.

The rot really set in, I suppose, when I was thirteen. In the space
of one school year I went from 8 stone 10 pounds (122 pounds) to 11
stone 7 pounds (161 pounds). Perhaps it was the suddenness of the
weight gain which made it hard to adapt. It's impossible to list all the
reasons – name-calling, the horrors of PE, not having a proper school
uniform (because blouses only went up to a size 36 bust).

Also, my mother blamed me for being fat. Phrases leap to
mind all the time. 'You could be pretty if you tried . . . You're
just doing it to annoy me.' Constant nagging. Knowing that I
embarrassed her.

I remember the near-impossibility of getting anything to wear!
(We're talking about the mid-seventies to early eighties.) Constant
self-consciousness – did it show that my bra was too small? Having
to wear my jersey all summer term because my school blouses didn't
fasten. Wearing lumpy acrylic skirts. Having no social life because I
literally had nothing to wear. I managed to cobble together something
for school (e.g. a man's white shirt, a couple of men's jerseys,
a waterproof cagoule from a camping shop, a mail order skirt)
and perhaps one or two other skirts for after school. The most
difficult thing was summer. There were just no clothes for summer –
perhaps a couple of cotton T-shirts – so I spent the summer holidays
indoors.

I was twenty-three before I was asked out on a date, and I did blame it on my size. However, I'm very happy with my present partner and have been for the past three years.

My mother is a diabetic and has been all of my life. A constant threat levelled at me throughout my childhood and youth was, 'If you don't lose weight you'll end up diabetic like me.' Of course as a child I never had the courage to say, 'But you're thin, Mum, so why are you diabetic?' She also told me when I was six that 'Fat children grown up to have twisted bones.' And there were all the other health threats of flat feet, varicose veins and heart attacks. I went through a phase in my early teens when I lived in dread of having a heart attack. Consequently I have always tended to be afraid of doctors.

A couple of years ago I injured my shoulder in an accident and couldn't pluck up courage to ask for treatment because I guessed I'd have to be referred to hospital for physiotherapy – although I have a great GP who has never suggested I lose weight. (I have heard on the grapevine that she used to be involved with a self-help group for women with eating disorders. I am hanging on to my wonderful GP at all costs!)

I don't have any happy memories of food. When I was a young teenager I would come home from school and my mother would present me with some dieting gimmick (e.g. Carnation Slender meal replacements, or those toffee food replacements called Aids) and inform me that I had to use it. It was such a slap in the face. I always felt like such a failure. Such a disappointment.

One of the most searing memories of my food problems comes from my university days. I used to eat my packed lunch in a toilet cubicle because I wasn't able to eat in front of other people. One day I noticed that my particular cubicle had sweet papers and food wrappers strewn all over the floor. 'Geez,' I thought, 'I'm not the only one.'

My general strategy is to do my best to make sure that being fat is the only problem (if it *is* a problem) that my body has to deal with. I have never smoked, don't drink, eat very well and exercise regularly. I swim about four or five times a week, learned to cycle when I was twenty-six and do a bit of hill-walking.

Linda's story highlights how a little knowledge can be very dangerous. By reading about dieting in a teenage magazine she learned that dieting was 'normal'. Her experiences and Joan's emphasize the need for size awareness sessions, especially for people who work with children. Finally, I wish I had a pound for every time I've heard people complain about lack of clothes choice.

Mandie

Height 5 foot 10 inches Weight 12 stone (168 lb) Age: Twenty-two
Occupation Factory worker

My one wish is to be able to forget dieting and stop worrying about my body size. I have been dieting non-stop for as far back as I can remember. My mum has always dieted too, and so after I received a few jokes about my size at school I decided I would follow suit.

I began to get paranoid, and one of my earliest memories of how miserable worrying about your body size was is quite funny. I was in the junior school (so I was younger than eleven) and besotted with horses, like a lot of young girls at that age. The walls of my room were covered in horse posters and religiously, every night before I got undressed, I would pull the top two pieces of Blue-Tak from the wall so that the horses' heads faced towards the wall and they couldn't see my body as I undressed! Then before I got into bed every poster was put back up again. This ritual was repeated for years.

Until recently, dieting has just been a part of my life. Every Monday I began a new diet, and it became a standing joke to everyone who knew me. I was the butt of many jokes, and the lads in the factory in which I work were the worst. Laughingly, I would answer them back and put myself down to show that it didn't bother me. But in actual fact, every time they joked about my size it was like someone had stabbed me.

I was confused and hurt by their attitudes. At 5 foot 9 inches and weighing about 12 stone, I was not 'huge'. I didn't like myself, but I didn't regard myself as huge and I still wore size 14 clothes. But if someone tells you often enough you start to believe it. I don't think I helped myself by laughing along with them, but I didn't know what else to do.

Anyway, I got more and more miserable and tried more and more diets. With each one I lost weight initially, but after sticking to it for a short while I put on everything I had lost plus some more. I got heavier and heavier until I reached 13 stone (182 pounds) and hit rock bottom. I became very depressed and would cry for no reason at all.

I blamed my husband of less than a year for my moods, and on a number of occasions I planned to leave him. He was an absolute hero and stood by me the whole time, even though I hurt him badly with the things I said.

I became dirty – not washing my hair, not cleaning my teeth, and in general just not giving a damn about my appearance because I wasn't going anywhere. Going out became really hard for me, as I was ashamed of myself and couldn't bear to be seen in company.

Finally, it got too bad and I became suicidal. Every time I was on my own and feeling down, I would plan what I could do. The best move I made was to tell my sister, and she came with me to the doctor's. The doctor sat and talked to me for an hour and a half. Since then I have been seeing her weekly and have had counselling. As a result I have come to realize why I was depressed about my body size and the pressure to be slim.

We keep narrowing the goal posts . . . Mandie was size 14 and getting hurtful remarks aimed at her. Reading Mandie's story I was reminded of the frozen peas advert, where only the tiniest peas get through the gates. The 'truth' is that, whatever our size, none of us is good enough . . . we are all *fat*. And for 'fat' read 'revolting'.

Angela

Height 4 foot 11 inches Weight 8 stone (112 lb) Age Thirty-five Occupation Not supplied

As a very young child I didn't have problems with weight, but from the age of about eleven I began to put it on. At thirteen I started to diet. I remember my aunt saying she was going to Weight Watchers, and I thought I could lose some weight on my own.

I did lose quite a few pounds (I don't recall what my weight was at that stage). However, by the time I was seventeen and in my last year at school I was 9 stone 7 pounds (133 pounds). I was too heavy for my height, it sapped my confidence, I was a shy person anyway and it seemed to ruin everything. I never felt 'part of' anything – I was always on the outside of a group. I did have a few friends, but they were mostly quiet ones, like myself.

I never suffered from anorexia but my eating habits were far from sensible – often surviving on an apple, a few crispbreads, and maybe some nibbles of chocolate etc. which I felt didn't count. I was on and off the scales (I still am) and would often rush home from college and demolish half a dozen slices of bread and jam because I was so ravenous.

Towards the end of college, when I was twenty-one and about to start training as a solicitor, I had managed to get my weight down to about 8 stone (112 pounds). I began to feel much better about myself and remembered thinking, 'I'll lose a few more pounds and then stop!'

However, the pattern of not eating sensibly continues, with bingeing sessions which often happen on a Friday evening after work. One day when I was about twenty-five I really did 'pig out'. I felt so full and uncomfortable that I thought, 'If I could be sick I would feel better.' I stuck my fingers down my throat.

After this episode I felt disgusted with myself and vowed never to do it again. But a few weeks later I did, and then gradually it became a regular habit two or three times a week.

I worked out a way to lose weight – I ate hardly anything until mid-afternoon, and then binged until I arrived home. I would have supper about 6pm with my parents and sisters (I would eat a light meal – I was too full to manage anything else) and then disappear upstairs and make myself sick.

At first I refused to accept that there was anything the matter with me. I could eat what I wanted *and* lose weight. But I did worry that I could be doing myself internal damage.

One day – I can't remember the actual occasion – I read an article about bulimia and realized I must be suffering from it. From then on I read everything I could about this disease in an effort to scare myself to stop. At the age of twenty-eight, a few months before I was due to be married, I managed to stop. The seriousness of what I was doing to myself finally dawned.

Unfortunately the bulimia returned some six months later, and for some reason my willpower snapped about every six months when I had just the one attack.

It finally stopped two and a half years ago, and since then I have felt 100 per cent in control, with no urge to make myself sick. However, I cannot accept my shape and weight as they are. I am not fat. I am totally fed up with dieting and would love to throw out the scales and my too tight clothes, but after years of dieting it's hard to change the habits of a lifetime.

Angela's story shows how easy it is to slip from dieting into a more serious eating disorder. At thirteen Angela would have been growing into womanhood. We need to let girls know that it is right that their bodies are getting bigger – not just on an individual, personal basis, but as a society. We need to celebrate images of womanhood of all ages and sizes rather than revere the flat-chested, narrow-hipped young boy look – which only 5 per cent of the female population can ever attain.

Carole

Height 5 foot 1 inch Weight 12 stone (168 lb) Age Forty-seven Occupation Not supplied

I have been unhappy with my body since I was thirteen years old. Now I'm forty-seven, and I'm still unhappy, if not more so. My whole life has revolved around wanting to be thin.

When I was in my teens I weighed about 8 st 7 pounds (119 pounds), which, looking back, was OK for my height and sturdy frame (size 6 shoe). But even then I felt that I was too fat, and I started to diet at the age of sixteen.

Since I had my twins Kate and Alex, now ten, I have put on about 3–4 stone (42–56 pounds). I have tried everything: hypnosis, acupuncture, exercise, diet clubs, Cambridge diet – you name it, I've had a go at it. It's foolishness really, but I keep hoping that I will find the 'magic' formula.

I have held back from people and places because I never felt that 'chubby little me' looked good enough, and I thought that everyone else noticed what a fatty I was. Sad that a woman of my age has let life pass her by because she always feels too 'fat' to get out there in the 'real' world and take a few risks.

The DB questionnaire

Our need to be dieting and constantly watching our weight hasn't just sprung up from nowhere. I designed the DB questionnaire to help women gain insight into their relationship with their bodies, food and dieting, and to discover how this may be related to other things in our lives – both past and present.

My hope is that by identifying patterns we can begin to understand why we do things, and that this understanding will help us stop brutalizing ourselves – with the diet mentality and self-loathing.

Please make sure you answer questions 14 and 15.

1. Have you ever wished you were thinner? If so, by how much?

2. What have you done about it?
3. What/who has stopped you/how have you stopped yourself from accepting yourself as you are?
4. Have you ever felt any pressure to diet from others? If so, list in order of 1, 2, 3 etc. where the most pressure has come from:
   Partner ( ) Children ( ) Mother ( ) Father ( ) Friends ( ) Colleagues ( ) Doctors ( ) The Media ( ) Advertising ( ) Fashion Industry ( ) Other . . .
5. Describe one bit of pressure you have experienced about your body/size/shape/weight/appearance generally.
6. How did you deal with it?
7. Describe any negative feelings you have/have had about (a) yourself generally (b) your body in particular. Be specific about which parts of your body.
8. Write a brief history of your relationship to food.
9. Describe one happy and one unhappy memory you have about food/eating/dieting in your childhood.
10. If you have ever dieted, which diets have you tried and what were the results?
11. Approximately how much money have you spent on slimming/ diet products, foods, books, clubs, videos etc.?
12. Specifically in relation to you building greater self-esteem and confidence:
    (i)   what/who has helped, and how?
    (ii)   what/who has hindered, and how?
    (iii) can you think of anyone who might help, if you asked?
13. Did/does your mother diet? Has her relationship with food affected you? If so, how?
14. What is your nicest physical attribute?
15. List two of your personal qualities.

What was that like to complete? What did you feel as you were answering the questions? Writing things down can really bring ideas and feelings to the surface in a different way from just verbalizing them. Many women told us that answering these questions really helped them to make connections between their relationship with food, their bodies and their past experiences.

Give yourself time to think about your replies. You may gain some insights or be able to make connections between your experiences and feelings.

3

Take It with a Pinch of Salt

What you really lose

The diet industry is laughing all the way to the bank. Annual turnover in the USA is $33 billion, making it the country's fifth largest industry, and even in the UK the turnover is £1 billion a year. It is the perfect product – it promises so much, and when it doesn't deliver the consumer blames herself and then goes on to the next diet. As one investment banker told *Newsweek*, 'We see tremendous potential. Our goal is to McDonaldize weight loss.'

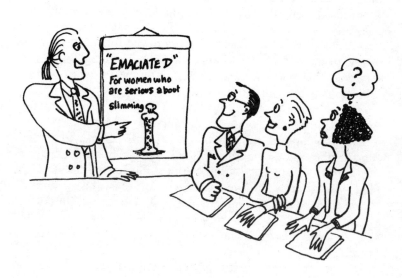

If you've been on a diet, lost weight and then regained it, it's not because there is something wrong with you. It's not because you have no willpower, are a failure or lack moral fibre, and it's not as if women today are ignorant about nutrition and the calorific value of different foods. So what's the problem? Why aren't we more successful? Why can't we diet and lose weight permanently? Fundamentally:

- We are not able to integrate diet behaviour into our normal lifestyle because it is abnormal
- We are fighting against our body's natural regulatory mechanisms
- Dieting is based on guilt, deprivation and sacrifice, which are difficult to sustain
- We are responding to external cues which don't address underlying issues
- We lose touch with our natural hunger signals

However, as with smokers who know that smoking can damage their health, there is always someone one who can tell a story about their Aunty Flo who got through forty fags a day and lived to be 104. And many dieters are the same – fingers crossed, ever hoping that they will be the exception to the rule, that they will be one of the 4 in 100 for whom diets work. No gambling woman would lay their money on such odds, but a dieter would.

And that's another of the ways in which diets hook us. They encourage us to believe we will be exceptional, lucky, different from the others, successful, better, and it's oh-so-easy.

This is a sample of the language of simplicity: 'quick and simple', 'slim for life', 'lose weight fast', 'think slim', 'thin think', 'guaranteed inch loss', 'slim fast', 'Chinese slimming secret', 'flush fat right out of your arteries', 'rub your stomach away', 'natural preparation which digests fat', 'the one-day diet', 'slim-patch weight control system', 'FB900 Fat Breaker Miracle Diet Capsules', 'sleep and slim capsules', 'size 12 in 21 days', 'outsmarting the female fat cell'.

Women feel good for just having made the decision to go on a diet. Weight loss is a challenge, it's exciting, and there is a sense of achievement as the pounds fall off. Admiring glances, compliments and the ability to wear fashionable clothes can be glorious bonuses. For many it becomes a hobby and a social activity. As a Weight Watchers leaflet says, 'Success is just one step away.' Just take one step over the mat and even the ugliest of ducklings will, magically and effortlessly, be transformed into a beautiful swan whom everyone loves and admires.

The downside is the feeling of living on a knife edge, that you are only one bite away from failure, that you're a fraud because you need to put in so much effort to be this attractive – you can't achieve it naturally. Then, when you start putting the weight back on, you feel a failure. 'Oh, you've put on weight, haven't you? Poor you!'

Feeling fat is something that most women know. It has become a quick and easy way to describe horrible feelings. Many diets promise almost instant success or relief – and here is another hook. Focussing on our weight and then going on a diet may seem to serve a useful purpose. It may appear to offer a solution to other, deeper problems. By going on a diet you are at least doing something to get rid of those horrible feelings. The tragedy is that if we simply take the short cut in describing our feelings as 'fat', and look for the instant solution to this problem, we may never learn and understand the true nature of our feelings or develop strategies to deal with them effectively.

When the diet mentality takes hold of us we stand to lose a lot more things than the hoped-for weight. The goal of becoming thin can cause us to suspend our common sense. We believe any Jack-the-Lad's promises, whether they are peddling seaweed patches, beans-in-a-bag smelling of chocolate (to stop you eating it, apparently, though I thought the point of using a pleasant fragrance was to encourage us to want more) or papaya pills purporting to be fat busters.

Dieting calls for sacrifices. Sacrifices are neither easy nor natural – which is, I believe, another reason why so many dieters give up. Deep, deep down we are not prepared to sacrifice ourselves on the altar of narcissism. On the other hand, that feeling of self-sacrifice can hook us into wonderful feelings of purity and goodness.

To be a successful dieter you have to stick religiously to the regime, be constantly vigilant and, as a result, become inward-looking. Ask yourself whether you would choose to share a glass of wine and break bread with someone who is obsessed with calorie counting – or to live day in, day out with food and dieting as the main topic of conversation.

The diet becomes a kind of fanatical religion, requiring you to abide by a set of stringent rules or pay the penance of guilt. It's a guilt that starts by slowly nibbling and then steadily gnaws away at your body, spirit and confidence. Give yourself a break. You deserve much, much more.

Until now the diet mentality has reigned supreme. It has become such an acceptable part of our culture and our lives that we don't even ask 'Why?' when we hear that a person is on a diet. And we don't ask 'Why not?' when a product doesn't seem to be working.

Some women feel more guilty about cheating on their 'eating plan', as the industry now call their diets, than they do about fiddling their income tax return or cheating on their partner. As a dieter, you are part of the mainstream and yet you are out of it. This letter to Diet Breakers from Josie says it all,

It would be wonderful not to feel 'different' from the rest of humanity – but dieting makes people feel like that: full of guilt, seeing ourselves as much fatter than we really are, 'naughty' for eating things we shouldn't, and not being able to feel secure without actually dieting. It's a vicious circle which is time-consuming and at times expensive, and both physically and psychologically damaging to our health.

We are hooked into believing it is desirable to be thinner than we are, whatever our size, and never to be satisfied with the way we are. And the 'good news' from the dieting industry is that a desirable weight and body are achievable by 'cheat eating' their miracle products so that 'we won't even feel like we are dieting'. We'll think about, and plan for, the time when we are thinner – and then we are terrified that we won't be able to sustain it. So you hang on to your large clothes, because you never know when you're going to need them.

You pays your money . . .

So what are you getting when you hand over your money to a diet plan or product? Fiona gave birth to her first child and immediately afterwards was very anxious to get back to her original weight and shape. She said she was not really able to enjoy being pregnant because she couldn't separate being pregnant from being fat, which for her meant being unattractive.

She wanted to lose 10 pounds, so she joined a ten-week scheme which included 'counselling' sessions, a workbook and a range of food products. She lost the weight but, alas, started to regain it shortly afterwards when she began to eat proper food again. She had given away almost £1000 on fees and special food, together with the joy of new motherhood.

Jennifer was a student who got a holiday office job with the Cambridge Diet. Under her terms of employment she was to receive free supplies of the diet and be the shop window mannequin shedding pounds before the customers' eyes.

The diet works by fooling your body into thinking you are in a state of starvation. Jennifer was consuming fewer than 500 calories a day; as a result her body went into a state known as ketosis, which occurs during starvation or when people are on a low carbohydrate diet. What happens is that the body mobilizes fat tissue to make substances called ketones which are used for energy instead of the normal glucose. The ketones can be smelt on your breath (some people say it reminds them of pear drops), and this is a sign that your body is trying to maintain a balance in the face of extreme deprivation. If your body didn't react in this way at such times, you would die. After three highly uncomfortable days of starvation, weakness, light-headedness and headaches, Jennifer's brain shut off the hunger signals. The clock was her only reminder that it was time to eat.

On the Cambridge Diet, breakfast, lunch and dinner each consisted of a glass of strawberry, vanilla or chocolate milk shake. Jennifer says she worked long hours at the diet centre, advising women of all shapes and sizes – but mostly comparatively slim women – how to take this powdered miracle. She stressed the importance of drinking eight pints of fluids a day – black coffee, diet cola or water – and told them never to go too far from the loo, because the milk shakes have a diuretic effect.

Back at home, Jennifer watched her family eat and thought, as she wrote to Diet Breakers: 'How obscene and uninitiated these people were, who ate by putting chunks of food into their mouths and chewing them!' Jennifer says she and the diet participants felt privy to some great secret. Telling people how well she felt helped to reinforce the message and the hook of helping her to

feel better than, and different from, other people. The wonderful
secret and the special preparations that 'shakers' undergo becomes
a purity ritual.

How did it end for Jennifer? As the summer waned, she began to
wake in the night with agonizing leg cramps. She asked for time off
work to visit the doctor, mentioning the reason to her employers.
She was told by a Registered Cambridge Diet Counsellor, 'Oh,
that's a regular symptom – you are a classic case.' She thinks the
cramps could have been caused by having been on the diet for
4–5 months, whereas most customers were on it for a matter of
weeks. When at the end of the summer vacation she returned to
college her love affair with food was rekindled, as was her love of
life, and, she says, 'As I further progressed with counselling and
personal development, my love of myself, with gently increasing
girth, started for the first time. Looking back I feel a cold shiver.'
Jennifer lost 5 stone (70 pounds), and regained it all.

In the early 1970s a new high protein, low carbohydrate diet
swept America. Over one million hardback copies alone were sold
of *Dr Atkins' Diet Revolution*. By the time the paperback version
was published, Dr Robert C. Atkins had been called to give
testimony before the US Senate Select Committee on Nutrition
and Human Needs. Certain charges had been made against the
diet by the American Medical Association and others, involving the
possibility of adverse effects to dieters' health. Dr Atkins' reply to
the Select Committee, on 12 April 1973, included these words.

Because every diet – like every medication, vaccination, surgical
innovation or other medical advance – is potentially dangerous if
misapplied, I have always recommended medical examinations and
blood tests before and during various stages of my diet or any other.
Symptoms of fatigue, lethargy, dizziness and hunger can occur in any
diet; but the American Medical Association is ironically correct in
stating that anorexia, or loss of appetite, is a side-effect of my diet.

This did not stop the publication of the paperback version
of the book. The publishers adroitly circumvented the 'minor'
setback with a publisher's note emphasizing the importance of
medical supervision prior to and during the diet. But what percentage of dieters consult their doctors before embarking on a
new diet?

The truth about diet foods

Considering how important food is to our overall good health, it seems mad that our choices may be motivated and determined by a catchy advertising jingle, current fad or the promise of a low calorie count (omitting to say lower than what – a Mars bar?). Under Britain's current health rules and regulations anything can call itself a diet product so long as it has the wording in brackets on the side of the packet, 'only as part of a calorie-controlled diet'.

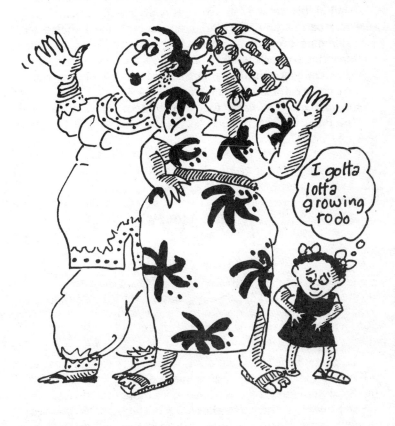

Sue Dibb and Juliet David from the Food Commission, together with Suzanne Owen of the Coronary Prevention Group, have researched meal replacements such as biscuits, bars and milk shakes, and other so-called healthy ready-made meals. None of the products came out very favourably, and most of them are far from healthy.

Generally speaking, the bars and mixes got the thumbs down for:

- *Causing people to lose weight too quickly*: cutting back too severely on calories can cause loss of lean tissue and a lowering of the metabolic rate
- *Poor nutrition*: most products were high in fats and/or sugars, and all biscuit and bar products were low in protein
- *Not being lower in calories*: in general, meal replacement slimming products were not significantly lower in calories than many snack foods
- *Encouraging unhealthy eating habits*: because of their emphasis on sweet and often high fat snacks
- *Selling less for more*: for their content, meal replacement products are expensive

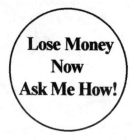

Lose Money Now Ask Me How!

The ready-made meals did not fare much better. Current health advice for everyone, and that includes dieters, is to increase our intake of complex carbohydrates and fibre and to cut down on salt and fats. It would therefore be reasonable, you would think, to assume that foods which describe themselves as healthy ready-made meals would adhere to these principles. Reasonable, yes – but not the case.

- A substantial number of the meals tested fell short of the Coronary Prevention Group targets. Most only scored marginally better than their ordinary counterparts
- Only 53 out of 75 meals gave nutritional information on saturated fat
- All the products in the survey scored high for salt
- Only 25 of the 75 meals met Coronary Prevention Group targets for fibre
- Just 59 per cent met the recommended level for carbohydrates

The Food Commission criticizes food manufacturers for not doing enough to help consumers eat less fat. A survey of reduced and low fat foods in leading supermarkets, which the Commission conducted in October 1994, found that manufacturers were charging up to 40 per cent more for lower fat equivalent products, and were failing to provide a wider range of lower fat foods. The survey found that:

- Wall's Too Good To Be True ice cream was 27 per cent more expensive than the same company's Gino Ginelli brand
- Tesco Healthy Eating burgers were 32 per cent more expensive than their regular beefburgers
- McVitie's Light Krackawheat was 33 per cent more expensive than their regular Krackawheat
- Findus Lean Cuisine chicken and pasta frozen ready meal was 40 per cent more expensive than Findus regular chicken lasagne

The report's author, Peta Cottee, said, 'Charging a premium cannot simply be explained by different ingredients. We found a few companies, such as Marks & Spencer and Ambrosia, offering ready meals and desserts in both regular and low fat versions at the same price.'

In 1992 consumers were promised tough new regulations by the Ministry of Agriculture, Fisheries and Food (MAFF) on low fat claims by food manufacturers. 'Low fat' would have to mean less than 5 per cent fat and less than 5 grams of fat in a typical serving. 'Reduced fat' would have to mean that the total fat content must be less than three-quarters that of similar products that make no claims. 'Fat-free' would have to mean that less than one-sixth of

1 per cent of the content was fat. The use of the word 'very', as in 'very low fat yogurt', would not be permitted.

But the proposals went down like a lead balloon with the food manufacturers, because many of their products would fail the new guidelines for fat content. MAFF have now gone cold on the idea, and the European Commission too have stalled. Furthermore, the word 'lite' is also still used freely for any of the following: reduced fat, calories, salt, sugar, alchohol and even colour. It is so misleading that it should be outlawed.

As an example of how the marketing of food products preys on our feelings of guilt, consider the behaviour of two supporters to Diet Breakers, Christine and Joanna. Christine would stock up her cupboards with crispbreads and low calorie spreads and an impressive array of dietary products. Then, slowly and determinedly, she would work her way through them. She would tell herself that she could eat a lot precisely because they were meant to assist her in dieting. Deep down she knew she could not justify eating the entire contents of a packet of crispbreads in one sitting and still claim she was on a diet – but for quite a while she did just that because it seemed to relieve her guilt about not dieting.

I saw something similar with Joanna, a student, who would order a packet of crisps and a diet drink. Her mother pointed out the contradiction in a packet of crisps and a diet drink. Joanna explained, 'I'm thirsty, so I want a drink, and I fancy a packet of crisps. I've ordered the diet drink so that I don't feel guilty about eating the crisps.'

Slimming clubs and their leaders

The diet mentality is perpetuated in dieting and slimming clubs where weight loss is cheered and congratulated amongst members. I leave it to you to ponder how the members who don't get clapped and cheered must feel. Motivation through humiliation?

In Britain there are approximately ten thousand diet club leaders. It is believed that only about one in ten members of clubs reach their target weight. The clubs claim they are providing a legitimate service by offering healthy nutritional advice. First you are weighed, then you are given a target weight and a recommended eating plan to help you achieve your goal. A lifetime membership is the prize if you reach and sustain your target weight.

I do not deny the usefulness of regular group meetings, the chance to meet and chat, to share experiences and failures and to get that often-needed pat on the back (which perhaps we are not getting elsewhere in our lives). But the groups' very names give them away: Slimming Magazine, Weight Watchers and, for the globally ambitious, Slimming World. They are in the business of weight loss. They have a vested interest in encouraging you to be dissatisfied with your body, to compare yourself constantly with other women, and to believe you do not possess the skills to make your own healthy lifestyle decisions.

They start off with the assumption that there is something wrong with you. By definition they are the experts and have the answers to your problems. All problems are defined in relation to weight:

- High weight = big problems
- Low weight = no problems
- No weight loss = your problem!

To my knowledge, no organization offers a refund when its regime fails you.

Typically, organizations recruit their group leaders from their more successful customers. It makes good business sense. The thin leader is there to remind us each week that some people do actually manage to get through the hoops and barriers and lose weight.

I have received a number of letters from women who used to run dieting clubs. They tell me their lives were hell because they lived in fear of losing their jobs. Some dieting club leaders are weighed every month, and if they have gained more than a certain amount of weight they are sacked. One woman from Yorkshire told me that induced vomiting for several days before the weigh-in is common amongst diet club leaders, and she knows of several who are fully fledged bulimics. Rather like the farm labourer's tied cottage arrangement, where his home is tied to his job, here we have the tied body.

Josie was a successful diet club leader for many years. In her heyday she organized several groups of seventy or eighty women each week, all coming to be weighed by Josie and to listen to her caring advice. But eventually she ditched her (very lucrative) job because she felt a fraud. She noticed that many of her 'ladies' returned again and again. With Josie's help they would get their weight down, and then a few months later back they would come, the weight regained, for another ride on the merry-go-round. Roller-coaster is a more apposite term, because that is what dieting feels like – a slow uphill struggle to get to a target weight, a feeling of exaltation at having reached the top, a quick look round at the view, and then *whoosh* . . . full speed downhill all the way back to the starting weight, and probably overshooting it and putting on a bit more.

Another person who couldn't control his weight was Richard Weston. He and his wife Bernice introduced Weight Watchers to Britain from America in 1967. Apparently they had both been 'overweight'; Bernice, for instance, was 5 foot 2 inches tall and weighed 14 stone (196 pounds). They started their new enterprise with just three members in the village hall at Datchet in Buckinghamshire. It prospered so well that in 1978 the Westons sold Weight Watchers to the multi-national company Heinz. Bernice told *Woman* magazine, 'Richard forced me to sell the business. I think it was partly for the money, but also because he wanted me out. He couldn't control his weight and was under constant scrutiny as a partner in Weight Watchers.'

Well, if Mr Weight Watcher himself couldn't keep his weight down, what chance do the rest of us have? Unfortunately, this is not easy to answer. Jane Ogden, says in *Fat Chance, The Myth of Dieting Explained*, 'A survey carried out in Britain suggests that about one in ten members of slimming clubs such as Weight Watchers and Slimming Magazine reach their target weight. However, it is difficult to understand what these figures actually mean. The clubs do not keep any information as to the weights of these women initially so there is no way of knowing how much weight they had to lose to be regarded as successful.'

And to rub salt in the wound we have Dieter or Slimmer of the Year competitions. In these cattle parades we see the real 'Martha' standing jubilantly beside a cardboard cut-out of her previous self looking very miserable and dejected and usually wearing ill-fitting clothes. Or 'Pat' will be standing inside a pair of extremely baggy trousers, holding out the waistband and telling us, 'This is what I used to look like when I let myself go, before I took control of myself.' Spare a thought for the person who does weigh 30 stone, and imagine what impact these competitions may have. How would you feel if a cardboard cut-out of a person your size is held up with the unspoken message: 'Don't end up looking like this fat cow'?

Of course, we don't see many interviews with former Dieters of the Year who have regained the weight, and/or hear about the impact their experiences have had on them. These competitions have other messages for us, too. To the thin women who make up the bulk of the dieting club membership, the message is: 'Our dieter of the year lost 5 stone, so you can lose 5 pounds', or: 'If you don't keep on coming you'll lose control and end up like the cardboard cut-out.'

Fear of losing control is like fear of the unknown. It figures prominently in the minds of many dieters and is exploited to the hilt by the slimming industry. Fear of the unknown, such as shadows in a darkened room, can be frightening. However, I have found that shadows change shape and definition, and even disappear altogether, when I turn on the light and open my eyes.

Sherry Ashworth, author of the wonderfully funny book *A Matter of Fat*, noticed at her local dieting club that most of the women joining each week were, in fact, old members rejoining. To maintain club revenues, it is important to let lapsed members know they are not forgotten and to remind them that the door – and the cash box – is always open to them. Clubs use a variety of techniques such as phone calls, cards, letters and poems as little encouragements to rejoin the fold. Brenda wrote, 'I received a poem this morning from Slimming World which I joined last year for a short period, but every couple of months I get some form of reminder.'

Well, the ditty didn't lure Brenda back to Slimming World, but it proved a source of inspiration for DB supporter Liz Shepperd:

Greetings to all at Slimming World
And thank you for your letter,
But there have been changes in my life
And all for the better.

Although it did impress me
When I received your verse
I've realized you only make
My situation worse.

I used to think you'd make me thin,
But now I know you won't,
For ninety-six to ninety-eight
Per cent of diets don't.

You'd think, since people try so hard,
Success would be assured,
So doesn't that suggest to you
Your methods might be flawed?

It's the ideas of self-contempt
I've chosen to reject,
I'm going to live a different life
With healthy self-respect.

Now I know that dieting
Tends to make me blue,
You won't be seeing me again,
I've better things to do!

Diets don't work

One of the reasons that dieting doesn't work is that it undermines our normal regulatory eating mechanisms and causes us to over-eat – usually the first sign of the diet breaking down.

As we lose large amounts of weight, so our daily energy requirement drops as we have less weight to carry. Therefore we don't need to eat as much and our body learns to use the food more efficiently. Although this is a pain in the pinafore for a dieter, it makes sense to your body.

People have evolved over millions of years, and starvation has at times been a real threat to the survival of the human race. Our bodies have developed a brilliant system of dealing with excess food so that it can help us out whenever there is a food shortage. This surplus food is stored in our bodies as fat, which can later be oxidized to produce energy when we need it. As we reduce the amount of food we eat, our body prepares for the invasion on its store cupboard.

Metabolic rate – the speed at which your body transforms food into energy – is affected by slimming and dieting. When you eat less, the rate goes down to enable you to function using as little energy and stored fat as possible. Your metabolic rate doesn't know you are on an expensive, calorie-controlled diet. For all it knows, you could be stranded in the Australian outback and in need of all the support it can give you. After being on a diet for two weeks, your metabolic rate can drop by up to 20 per cent.

This will begin to explain why you may find it hard to lose weight – even if you are eating less food than normal – and why persistent dieters find losing weight harder and harder. By reducing your metabolic rate your body will not need to use its stored fat unless and until it is absolutely essential to do so.

So to be a successful dieter you would have to eat less, and less, and less, to compensate for your ever-decreasing metabolic rate. I have had letters from women who have dieted for years, telling me that they live on 500 calories a day – and still are not losing weight. Some famously thin women, such as Nancy Reagan, are renowned for their birdlike appetites. The more you diet the more you will have to cut down – or out. Dr Emily Fox Kales, Director of the Eating Disorders Clinic at McLean Hospital, at Harvard University, has been following an anti-diet approach since 1975. She has said, 'It was medically irresponsible for me to ignore the fact that I was harming patients I put on calorie-deficient diets.'

Who's in control?

Dieting increases the likelihood of over-eating because of the way it affects our moods and state of mind. In the 1950s, long before the current dieting trend took hold in the west, there was already evidence that dieting caused over-eating. In one study thirty-six men were put on a calorie-controlled diet. For twelve weeks they ate approximately half their usual amount of food and lost about a quarter of their original weight. During the diet these men became preoccupied with food, sometimes even stealing and hoarding it. Their ability to concentrate decreased and they became apathetic and depressed. After the twelve weeks they were told they could eat as they pleased. Many binged, ate continuously or reported a loss of control over their eating patterns.

Recognize yourself in any of that? Me too. Over-eating, increased preoccupation with food and feelings of loss of control are all too familiar to the millions of us who have made a career of dieting – the estimated 90 per cent of women who diet at some time in their lives.

Janet Polivy and Peter Herman, professors in the Psychology Department at Toronto University, have been studying dieting for almost two decades. In one of their now celebrated studies, female students were given one 7.5 oz milk shake, two 7.5 oz milk shakes, or none. Immediately afterwards they were given three diferent flavours of ice cream to eat. The experiment was presented as a study in connection with taste, not in relation to dieting or quantity eaten. The students could eat as much or as little as they wanted.

Unbeknown to them, the ice cream bowls were weighed before and after they had eaten. All eating was done in private to prevent the students becoming self-conscious and to avoid peer group pressure. After the experiment the students were divided into those who were dieting and those who weren't.

Polivy and Hermann discovered that the non dieters ate the least ice cream after two milk shakes, most ice cream after no milk shakes, and an amount in between after one milk shake. The dieters, on the other hand, ate more ice cream following one or two milk shakes than after no milk shakes at all.

The evidence here is of dieters losing control, which flies in the face of one reason we are persuaded by the diet industry to diet: fear of being out of control. You can take their promises of being in control with a pinch of salt. When we are dieting, the one thing we are not is 'in control', because we have handed all control over to the products, the group leaders and the books. We are, in effect, trying to control our bodies through our heads.

Sabotaging our brains – and worse

A study by Dr Mike Green and Dr Peter Rogers of the Institute of Food Research in Reading looked at two groups of students, fifty-five in the first and seventy in the second, a third of whom were dieting. Thirty per cent of the dieters were judged to be undernourished. The students were asked to spot a series of odd or even numbers on computer screens over long periods; all the dieters did worse than the non-dieters, with a significantly lowered ability to sustain attention. Also, their reaction times were a lot slower and their short-term memory inferior.

As Dr Green says, 'It is very worrying that these women were in a sense sabotaging their brains and that air traffic controllers, doctors, lawyers or students sitting their finals might be vulnerable to the adverse mental effects of dieting.' And unfortunately this scenario covers vast numbers of women, not just this small group of students. Drivers, machinists, VDU operators, teachers, cooks, mothers – indeed anyone for whom dieting is accepted as normal behaviour – are potentially at risk.

The researchers felt that the impairment was possibly due to a direct lack of nourishment to the brain, or that it was perhaps what is called a distraction effect: the dieters are so worried about their body image and their food that this takes away mental processing space from what they should concentrate on. I buy that. As any dedicated dieter knows, you have to concentrate on the diet all the time.

Many women become weak, depressed, nervous and irritable when they are trying to lose weight, and there is evidence that eating disorders often begin after a period of intense dieting. Yet there is a commonly accepted belief that pursuing thinness is the same as pursuing good health.

Janet Polivy has documented the following health complications directly attributable to weight loss:

- gallstones
- cardiac disorders
- fainting
- weakness
- fatigue
- both slowed and increased heart rate
- raised cholesterol levels
- anaemia
- gouty arthritis
- oedema
- headaches
- nausea
- hair loss and thinning hair
- hypertension
- diarrhoea
- constipation
- aching muscles

- abdominal pain
- raised uric acid levels
- intolerance of cold
- loss of lean tissue
- changes in liver function
- dry skin
- muscle cramps
- amenorrhoea (loss of periods) and decreased libido
- various complications when returning to a normal diet from a fasting one, for instance oedema, potassium deficiency, bile duct disorders and pancreatic problems
- death

Cut to the bone

It simply isn't possible through dieting and exercising to turn from a woman who is shaped like Roseanne Barr into one shaped like Vanessa Redgrave, or from a Hillary Clinton into a Brigitte Neilson – except, perhaps, with the aid of a surgeon's knife. It can be difficult to be thin all over and still have large breasts unless you have breast implants, which unfortunately many women are now resorting to. Contrary to advertising and fashion designers' hype, women are meant to have breasts, hips, thighs and tummies. Yet, sadly, so often these are the very areas that women say they like least in their bodies.

But even surgery would have limited 'success': America's first lady-political partner will never be 6 feet tall, so if her role model were Brigitte Neilson she can forget it!

If we take a cultural and historical perspective, everything gets turned on its head. In many countries around the world – the Middle East, parts of Asia and Africa – what is disparagingly called 'fat' in Western society is very much admired. There, full stomachs, chubby faces and chunky thighs and buttocks are considered beautiful (see cartoon p47). In Europe, for many centuries the majority of the population lived a relatively hand-to-mouth existence, and only the privileged few could afford enough to eat at all times. So being large was a sign of wealth – a status symbol – whereas being thin meant you were malnourished and poor. Language supported the positive values of being fat:

compare 'portly', 'stout' and 'majestic' with 'flabby', 'blubbery' and 'gross'.

As with cigarettes, so with dieting. As dieting becomes less profitable in the West, the major weight loss companies will intensify their marketing in the developing world.

A house divided

When I tell people I am against dieting I am usually asked why. My explanation inevitably includes the following, by now familiar, points:

- 96–98 per cent of dieters regain all weight loss within 2–3 years
- Yo-yo dieting is not good for our health (see page 57)
- The majority of women who are trying to diet are thin to start with
- The diet industry makes most of its money from thin women

After that I am asked, 'Well, what about people who are *really* fat? They can't be healthy. They've got to diet, haven't they?' But this question diverts the debate from the main issue, which is that all women are now defined and valued in terms of the 'ideal' painfully thin body. It is an issue which divides women against each other because of their varying size.

This book is about the pressures on all women to have an 'ideal' body. Our bodies are perceived as public property – up for scrutiny and debate, rather than a personal matter. Because we all have to be very thin, it stands to reason that the fatter ones amongst us will be pressured most. I believe that if we accept that even one woman should be oppressed for her body size and shape we are all oppressed by body size and shape – because that is the gauge by which we are all being measured.

'Dieting is healthy'

Another reason I hate the 'What about fat people?' question is this: it presupposes that fat or 'obese' people have never tried to diet and that it's their fault, when in fact most of them are veterans of many failed diets. According to research undertaken by Dr Judith Rodin, founder of the Eating Disorders Clinic at Yale University, fat people eat no differently from thin people. And those who ask this fatuous question usually also assume that *all* fat people are running a health risk because of their size and weight – and that the solution is to diet.

The health factor is constantly being dragged up as a means and justification for refusing health treatment, for rude remarks and behaviour and for outright prejudice – most of which goes unchallenged. The diet industry 'sells' health as a main benefit from dieting, and now, in the face of increasing evidence of health risks associated with dieting, it has started to jump on to the anti-diet bandwagon. Some companies have even come out in support of International No Diet Day. Low fat spread wouldn't melt in their mouths!

Let's take a look at body fat and see what it does and doesn't do for you. The word 'obesity' is widely used to describe any degree of 'excess' weight. Obviously, from the diet industry's point of view this is very useful, because if this is the measure, then any amount of flesh, by definition, requires 'treatment' (for 'treatment' read 'weight loss diet').

We know that the majority of women on diets want to lose 10 pounds or less. Any fat is believed to be undesirable. But women are naturally fatter than men – between 18 and 30 per cent of the weight of a healthy woman is fat. On average, women live four to five years longer than men yet Shelley Bovey says in *The Forbidden Body* that no study has reported a direct relationship between 'overweight' and death from all causes, or from coronary heart desease.

Fat is necessary for the following reasons:

- It forms the body's energy store
- It protects delicate organs
- It is a vital structural component of all body organs
- It is important in reproduction;
  - to become fertile and grow breasts a young woman needs between 15 and 18 per cent of her body to consist of fat
  - to ensure sufficient energy store to give birth
  - to provide an important store for the early stages of breast feeding

- It produces oestrogen, which protects women from heart disease and brittle bones

We all become confused and seduced by health and weight propaganda, and the industry is perceived to be offering us a public service. This results in the majority of us being conned into equating thinness with good health.

However, I believe that in our bid for body emancipation we do need to be straightforward:

- To deny that weight can be a problem seems to me to be as irresponsible as saying that it is automatically a problem
- Fat and thin are not necessarily an accurate gauge of good and bad health
- Weight *may* be a problem – when in conjunction with other health risk factors
- Given the poor success rate of diets, for those people who do have a health problem the answer is surely *not* to 'go on a diet'
- I advocate self-acceptance and self-respect, followed by gradual healthy lifestyle changes that suit the individual – rather than a regime of self-loathing, deprivation, binge and guilt, which are the ingredients of diets

Look at Mo Moreland from the Roly Polys, who is in her seventies and yet can do the can-can, high-kicking like a twenty-year-old. Dawn French throws herself around with graceful aplomb, while Astrid Longhurst teaches aerobics and does the splits. These are all big women whose energy levels could be the envy of many of their thinner sisters. It is important not to jump to conclusions which connect a person's health and weight. Each person needs to be considered both as an individual and as a whole person – taking into account their medical history, lifestyle, gender, genetics, age and so on – before reaching any conclusions.

We also blithely follow standard height/weight charts, but in fact these are nowadays increasingly being questioned. Height/weight charts did not come from God or even from someone in the medical profession. They were designed by the insurance industry, whose typical policyholders were white Caucasian males in their twenties and thirties, and few died before they were fifty. Insurance

companies found that those people who did die under the age of
forty were mainly fat men – so they weighted their premiums
accordingly.

Health and weight, facts and myths

So what is the truth about the health risks of too much weight and
the healthy advantages of slimming? Most researchers and health
professionals usually use the term 'obese' to describe a person
with a BMI (Body Mass Index) of 30 and over. BMI = weight
in kilograms divided by height in metres squared. For instance if
you weigh 9 stone (57.3 kg) and are 5 foot 4 inches (1.6 m) tall,
your BMI = $57.3 \div 1.6 \times 1.6 = 22.4$

In the USA obesity is defined as a body weight of 20 per cent
or more above stated ideal weight ranges (US Department of
Health, Education and Welfare, 1979). Professor Frances Berg,
editor of the professional *Healthy Weight Journal*, suggests that
the term should be used to define the point above which weight
or fat contributes to health risk. In *You Don't Have to Diet*, Tom
Sanders and Peter Bazalgette list the health risks according to
BMI thus:

BMI	Risk
Less than 18	Very high risk
18–20	Moderate risk
20–25	Average risk
25–30	Low risk
30–35	Moderate risk
35–40	High risk
40+	Very high risk

Sanders and Bazalgette say that the risk of developing medical
disorders such as diabetes, high blood pressure and gout is slight
until BMI exceeds 28, when it increases rapidly. It is unusual for
people who are morbidly obese (with a BMI greater than 40) not
to have medical problems. But these authors also say that 'obesity
on its own is not a factor for risk of heart disease in the absence
of raised blood pressure, raised cholesterol or diabetes'.

More recently it has been suggested that the waist–hip ratio

Body Mass Index table

Height (inches)	19	20	21	22	23	24	25	26	27	28	29	30	35	40
						Body weight (pounds)								
58	91	96	100	105	110	115	119	124	129	134	138	143	167	191
59	94	99	104	109	114	119	124	128	133	138	143	148	173	198
60	97	102	107	112	118	123	128	133	138	143	148	153	179	204
61	100	106	111	116	122	127	132	137	143	148	153	158	185	211
62	104	109	115	120	126	131	136	142	147	153	158	164	191	218
63	107	113	118	124	130	135	141	146	152	158	163	169	197	225
64	110	116	122	128	134	140	145	151	157	163	169	174	204	232
65	114	120	126	132	138	144	150	156	162	168	174	180	210	240
66	118	124	130	136	142	148	155	161	167	173	179	186	216	247
67	121	127	134	140	146	153	159	166	172	178	185	191	223	255
68	125	131	138	144	151	158	164	171	177	184	190	197	230	262
69	128	135	142	149	155	162	169	176	182	189	196	203	236	270
70	132	139	146	153	160	167	174	181	188	195	202	207	243	278
71	136	143	150	157	165	172	179	186	193	200	208	215	250	286
72	140	147	154	162	169	177	184	191	199	206	213	221	258	294
73	144	151	159	166	174	182	189	197	204	212	219	227	265	302
74	148	155	163	171	179	186	194	202	210	218	225	233	272	311
75	152	160	168	176	184	192	200	208	216	224	232	240	279	319
76	156	164	172	180	189	197	205	213	221	230	238	246	287	328

(the circumference of your waist at its narrowest point when your stomach is relaxed, divided by the circumference of your hips at their widest – where your buttocks protrude most) is a more consistent indicator of cardiovascular disease than weight. This theory recognizes the two typical shapes of 'apple' (where there is a concentration of fat above the waist and around the belly, as in most men) and 'pear' (where there is fat around the hips and buttocks, as in most women). For men there is increased risk with a waist–hip ratio above 0.95, and for women when it is above 0.80.

The physiological differences between men and women and the fact that most adults gain weight with ageing are not highlighted by the diet industry. Men have a higher risk of cardiovascular disease if fat is concentrated around the abdomen (pot bellies) and although obesity in men has increased from 6% to 13% over the last 10 years, rates of heart disease have fallen by between 30% and 35%. Most of the deaths from heart disease in women occur at a relatively old age. Sanders and Bazalgete say, 'The risk of several non-fatal disorders such as diabetes, gallstones, gout, varicose veins and osteoarthritis increases with being overweight, but the risks are much greater in the very fat than the plump'.

According to Sanders, the current wisdom is that you're in a low risk situation if your BMI is below 30, you are reasonably active eat a balanced diet, don't smoke and maintain a stable weight

The bottom line

It may be worthwhile for some people to lose weight but we have exaggerated and misinformed ideas of who those people are. Not a single long-term study has proven that losing weight extends life.

Researchers don't know why, but all the recent evidence shows that our bodies resist major weight changes either up or down, and that, whatever the mechanism is, it also allows our bodies to increase in weight as we get older. The Elsie Pamuk (Centers for Disease Control and Prevention) study and the Harvard Study (1988) found that:

• Men and women with a stable BMI of 25–30, and BMIs of 25 or less, had similarly low death rates

- Any significant weight change either up or down markedly increased the risk of death from heart disease

The Framingham Heart Study, conducted by the NIH Heart, Lung and Blood Institute in Framingham Mass., began in 1948 and was the first major prospective study of cardiovascular disease. One of its findings was that:

- Those whose weight fluctuated frequently had a 50 per cent higher risk of heart disease than those whose weight remained stable

What we do know is that the health industry has failed dismally in attempting to treat obesity by dieting. I would like to see all health professionals and researchers working in the field of obesity attend size awareness workshops. We live in such a fat-phobic society that it is hard for any of us to avoid absorbing some of the negative messages we receive about fat people. This is bound to have an effect on our relationships with fat people. The only way forward is to stop shaming people into weight loss diets and instead focus on the goals of a healthy lifestyle and self-acceptance.

Natural weight?

The jury is out as to whether or not there is such a thing as 'natural' weight. It is likely that our body defends a weight within fairly narrow parameters, and there is good evidence that a lifestyle which includes nourishing, healthy food and a moderate amount of exercise will do quite nicely. Check whether you are in a high-risk group (see tables on pages 64 and 65) and, if you are concerned, see a qualified health practitioner. The reality for most of us is to incorporate some form of regular physical activity into our lives (see Chapter 6), to change our eating patterns gradually so as to follow current best advice, and, last but not least, to learn to be comfortable with our bodies at a stable weight, whether higher or lower than our present one, which makes us 'fit' for the things we want to achieve in our lives.

Thousands of women are now coming out against dieting. Their numbers include television presenters Judy Finnigan and Mariella

Frostrup, whose move is to be welcomed and applauded: because they are high-profile women they risk comment and ridicule at any time. Judy Finnigan came out on her *This Morning* TV show, saying she had had enough of dieting. 'It's hard. None of them work, and so they aren't worth the effort.' Well done, Judy, but wouldn't the tabloid press make you sick? Next day's headline: 'Judy Fattigan, never be Thinnigan', along with old photographs of her relaxing on a beach in the Mediterranean in a bikini etc. *Yawn*.

Mariella Frostrup bravely wrote about her dieting experiences and failures in the *Sunday Times* following, and in support of, MP Alice Mahon's Ten Minute Rule Bill to regulate the diet industry:

'I'm embarrassed to admit . . . I've found myself embarking on a variety of miracle diets. A hospital plan for heart patients which did the rounds a couple of years ago promised the loss of ten pounds in three days by eating a combination of dried toast, tuna and steamed cauliflower in very precise quantities. Faced with such a ghastly combination, it was hard work eating at all, but I determinedly stuck to it and after three days found I'd lost one measly pound.

Next came the vodka and grapefruit diet, a far more pleasing prospect. This entailed drinking a pint of juice before every meal, which the authors maintained would devour the fat content, and then washing it down with as much vodka as I could handle. Not surprisingly I don't remember much about that one apart from the hangovers and the horror on the tenth day when I stepped on the scales and (predictably) discovered that I'd put on weight.

At one stage in desperation I consulted a doctor who prescribed the then little-known drug Prozac, which he maintained would see the pounds fall off. Two weeks later I'd lost nothing, but luckily, thanks to its anti-depressant qualities, felt quite content about it. This was swiftly followed by a four-week course of Slendertone, concentrating on my hips and thighs, at the end of which the only weight loss I could find was from my wallet.

I've now resigned myself to two things: I'll never be a waif and the only time I actually lose weight is when I'm under pressure and my nicotine and caffeine quota rises. This may not be the healthiest option, I agree, but I think the same can be said for most of the diet plans currently on offer.

At one level for dieters there is a positive feeling of taking control, of doing something proactive to change the way they are, to change their situation. Dieting can be symbolic; a spring cleaning or self-cleansing of the body and spirit towards a better self and a better life. It's another chance. Unfortunately, the vision can so easily crumble even when there are short-term 'successes' at weight loss. Belief in oneself and increased self-esteem come from more fundamental inner changes, not from achieving a thinner physique.

The other way of looking at it is that we are in fact giving away control to others: the diet industry, the food industry, the peddlers of false dreams. They are saying that we don't have the ability to manage our bodies and our eating. To an extent it's true: we have lost touch with the natural responses to our physical and emotional needs, so we think we have to rely on others to provide a magic cure.

But with awareness and knowledge we can start to respond in ways which are more likely to give us what we want and enable us to be happier. The rest of this book is about that.

4

Breaking Free: You Can Do It

'Freedom's just another word for nothing left to lose'
Kris Kristofferson

Ode to Dolores

Dolores Delaney – a Diet Breaking lady
Stands big and stands tall and stands proud.
There's no way that she'll diet
Creep round and stay quiet
She's bright and she's funny and LOUD.

Dolores Delaney – a Diet Breaking lady
Never says,
Oh my God, I'm a mess!
She says, Don't diet – do it
Take a big bite and chew it
Go out in the world and say YES!

Dolores Delaney – a Diet Breaking lady
Loves swimming and music and fun
She's a go-getting lassie
Inclined to be sassie
Who likes to live life on the run

Dolores Delaney – a Diet Breaking lady
Is fierce, independent and strong.
Be the best you can be!
Her philosophy
Whether small, fat, tall, thin, big or long!

Dolores Delaney – a Diet Breaking lady
Knows she's extra-special and great

She loves eating and movement
And some self-improvement
She lives life to the full – she won't wait!

Dolores Delaney – a Diet Breaking lady
Can't understand people who sit.
If only I lost weight . . .
My whole life would be great
Get out there, RIGHT NOW AND LIVE IT!

                                              Linda Taylor

Worthwhile goals

This chapter is the beginning of your on-going journey to a diet-free
zone. Knowing the harm it can cause, since 1991 I have been
suggesting that women stop dieting. However, I recognize from
personal experience that you need to feel relatively secure, not at
risk of being stranded or abandoned. To help you move forward,
you need to reduce the likelihood of a 'disaster' that would throw
you back into the diet mentality, and you need to prepare for the
setbacks that may occur along the way.
    The rest of this book aims to help you to:

- Acknowledge and celebrate your personal qualities, skills and
  abilities
- Increase your vitality and confidence through welcoming back
  and appreciating your body
- Develop a healthy relationship with food to give you the
  energy to get on with your life
- Enjoy the social pleasures of eating without feeling guilty
- Incorporate physical activity into your life for enjoyment – not
  punishment
- Establish measures of success for yourself that are not related
  to weight loss and body perfection
- Feel attractive in the way you present yourself to the outside
  world – a way which is self-determined and self-affirming
- Appreciate the beauty and qualities in other women

- Be healthy and happy
- Recognize, accept and feel comfortable with your personal power

Contrary to the diet industry's promises of the quick fix, diet emancipation is achieved from a number of different directions and over a period of time. Giving up dieting, like a resolution to give up smoking on a certain day of next week, is easy. But it will only be sustained by addressing the fundamental emotional issues behind it. At the end of the day only you can make the choice to stop dieting and to confront the barriers that are keeping you hooked in the diet cycle.

Towards the end of this chapter I will be suggesting that you stop dieting and put food in its proper place – as fuel to keep you going and as one of life's pleasures. By nourishing your 'physical' hunger you will be meeting a fundamental need of your body. When you begin doing this, you will be much better equipped to nourish yourself in other ways.

- Are you now ready to start taking responsibility for yourself and finding out what's right for you, instead of some 'off-the-peg' fake remedy?
- Can you accept that there is no 'magic' solution?
- Are you prepared to find out what you're really feeling and what you really want?
- Are you ready to ditch the diet?

Diet Breaking will free us from the diet mentality which holds us back, and will enable us to achieve a whole range of sustainable objectives:

- Reclaim your body and enjoy it!
- Appreciate your personal qualities and those of others
- Improve your wellbeing, both mental and physical
- Enjoy food and its social aspects without feeling guilty
- Improve your body image, and feel more attractive
- Get more out of life and fulfil your potential
- Enjoy being a woman – get in touch with your femaleness and sexuality

• Feel the power and the pleasure of being your own woman

I have set out the journey in a number of stages, but they don't necessarily happen in a logical order. They are designed to prepare you for the transition to non-diet, or 'normal' behaviour, whatever that means to you. The best approach for each stage is to work out your answer to the question: 'What can I positively do in this situation, however small, to effect my journey to a diet-free zone?' I call this being proactive, as opposed to reactive – which is more about responding to others or waiting for things to happen (you could wait forever). The more proactive and more heavily engaged in other activities you are, the greater your success is likely to be.

By exerting an influence, through our behaviour, on the various aspects of our lives, we start to build up confidence. There are some influences on us, like that of the slimming/food industry, that we cannot change overnight (more on this later); but equally there are many others that we can. Asking for support from our close friends, or exploring ways to increase our awareness of the tyranny of thinness, are two examples.

Begin with the areas of your life where you have some expectation of success. This will give you confidence. There's no point in going for your most fearful situation first and setting yourself up for early and predictable failure.

Wanting to do it

Why do you want to start the journey? You may feel just plain fed up with dieting. You may feel desperate and trapped. You may feel a failure after many unsatisfactory diets. And then there are the feelings of dissatisfaction – what am I missing? There must be something more to life. Is it all passing me by?

Susan, for instance, said, 'At least I feel I'm beginning to get to grips with myself. I have a daughter of eleven and I don't want her to end up like me – diet-crazy. So I have stopped being obsessed with what I eat. My main topic of conversation is no longer what I shall have for lunch today or what I ate for dinner last night.'

Jenny wrote,

I dieted constantly between the ages of seventeen and twenty-four, yo-yoing from eight to ten and a half stone. I even became bulimic for about six months. It seemed like an easy way to control my weight. I'm not sure what finally brought me to my senses: self-disgust and real fears about my health, probably.

I went to the USA, where the diet industry is huge. It could have been the all-pervading obsession with body shape (masquerading as health and fitness) that made me realize just how (un)important it is to have a fat-free body. I'm very worried about the numbers of people dieting and with eating disorders. What are the long-term effects on our health? I met women in America of my own age (twenty-seven) who have undergone major surgery to change their bodies and faces. Is this the next step for women in Britain?

It's true that my weight has stabilized since I gave up dieting. I don't know what I weigh, but I'm a size 12.

Judy, a woman of thirty-eight who had been dieting since she was nine, said that having her son made her realize that her priorities were all wrong. She knew now that there were more important matters in life than one's appearance.

Fiona said,

Towards the end of my forties I left my husband, my self-esteem in shreds through obsessional dieting. I thought I was no good for anything. I did return, and my husband and I ironed out many difficulties, both real and imaginary. Having reached rock bottom, the only way was up. I started and ran a ladies' club, got elected as a local councillor, and now think a lot better of myself.

For some of us an event will trigger what we've always known subconsciously, and enable us to see the light. I didn't see the light, but a little seed of hope was sown when one day my husband, Derek, asked me, 'Are you going to be doing this for the rest of your life?' This question wasn't enough to change my behaviour, but it did lead me on to thinking that perhaps I had another option, and that perhaps he would help me. It seems asinine to have imagined that he would not notice my strange relationship with food.

Denise had tried just about every diet going, and says,

The last one that stands out in my mind was not actually designed as a slimming diet, but for cellulite. I was on this exercise regime

for twelve months, running fifteen miles a week. Imagine my horror
when I came back from a holiday abroad and saw by the photos that
the cellulite had got worse. My knees were fatter than when I had
started.

This was five years ago, and after that I swore not to have anything
to do with dieting again. I had finally learnt my lesson and threw
everything to do with the diet programmes, supplement pills and
even an enema kit(!) into the bin.

So maybe we want to do it because we're not happy with our
current circumstances and we have an inkling that things can be
better. You want to be free to be yourself. You may already have
a vision of how things will be different, you see you will have a
greater sense of freedom, and you want to be more open in your
relationships. You want to be more flexible in your response to
situations and to seize opportunities. Perhaps you can see that in
the long term you will be more confident and want to achieve your
personal goals.

It is possible that you will feel a sense of loss or emptiness, and
we shall deal with these feelings later. At this stage it is important
for you to find positive reasons to want to break your diet habit:
wanting to do something different and believing you are worth the
effort, even if you don't feel it at the moment.

Believing it is possible

Since dieting is very hard, it is reasonable to assume that not dieting
must be easier. And it is, once you get started. But don't confuse
'non-dieting' with 'not dieting'. If you just decide not to diet for a
week or so, you will still be in the diet mentality. At the back of
your mind will be filed the old thought, 'Oh, well, if this doesn't
work I'll find something else . . .' You need to give yourself at
least six months, preferably a year, to measure your success. It
is much the same as a smoker who has not had a cigarette for
two weeks – if she were to light up today, she would probably
be back in the habit. You need to give your mind and body time
to settle into a new way of living. Believing it is possible helps,
as does the belief that you are intrinsically capable and worth
the effort.

You have reached a certain point in your life and have acquired skills, knowledge and abilities that have seen you through. We all have a long list of achievements to our name: you learned to speak, to read and write, to pass exams, to cook without killing yourself with salmonella; you cross the road safely every day, you are holding down a job, running a home, bringing up kids, helping in your community . . . and so on and so on. You have the ability and potential to learn and acquire new skills as and when necessary. By focussing on the negative experiences we can all too easily forget how much we have achieved so far in our lives. I would like you to validate your successes, however small, every step of the way – because success breeds success.

So make a point of noticing your successes. When you do something well, congratulate yourself. If you complete a project, stand back and admire your work. Take pride in your efforts and share them with people who will appreciate them. If you have difficulty remembering, write down your achievements at the back of this book or in your diary. If you are creative, display your work. If you have a photograph of you doing something that you are proud of, look at it and enjoy it, and show it to people.

Another method is to give yourself positive affirmations regularly. If you have never done this before it might seem really uncomfortable or embarrassing. Social conventions have conditioned us into being sparing with praise, in the belief that it causes 'big-headedness' in ourselves and others. I disagree: most people flourish through positive and constructive feedback.

Stop taking yourself for granted! When we are feeling low it can become almost impossible to find something positive. At this time you need to work that bit harder to find something good about yourself. Look at your list of achievements or enlist the help of your support systems (see page 85), rather than reach for a diet product with its empty promises of quick relief. If you are feeling very low for a period of time and have no one whom you feel you can ask to help you out, seek professional help from a trained therapist or counsellor.

These are just a few ideas. It doesn't matter how you do it, just so long as you are validating yourself.

Another useful aid to help you get going is to select a role model:

in this case someone who has liberated herself from 'bodyism', who projects a positive image of herself and gets on with her life without necessarily being size 8 or dressing like a fourteen-year-old. If she does happen to be size 8 she will not be making a big deal of it or suggesting that she attained success simply by being that size. And she definitely will not be seen advocating a diet or eating plan on the front covers of women's magazines.

No one looking for a role model needs to look further than the magnificent black writer and singer Maya Angelou. For middle-aged women Bea Arthur from *The Golden Girls* is a brilliant role model, and it is inspiring to hear fashion model Lauren Hutton, a naturally thin woman who is in her fifties and still working, insist that advertising agencies who want to use her must take her as she is. She refuses to have cosmetic surgery or to allow photographers to retouch her wrinkles. Teresa Gorman, MP for Billericay, has built a successful career for herself after entering Parliament in her late fifties. We tend to think of most actresses, especially young ones, as glamorous, because that's the image of themselves they usually present. Helena Bonham Carter would seem to be no exception – yet she is definitely her own woman, and says she wears Doc Martens with everything by choice, simply because she wants to feel comfortable.

Many other women in the public eye have developed their own image without reference to any stereotyped 'ideal': Tessa Sanderson, Betty Boothroyd, Diane Abbott, bell hooks, Brenda Emanus, Kathryn Franklin, Josette Simon, Vanessa Feltz, Germaine Greer and Alison Moyet are just a few examples, and you can probably think of lots more. Dawn French, who always looks good and has certainly found her own style, has been an inspiration to many women. Sheena told me, 'After seeing Dawn French on television I went out and bought a costume and went swimming for the first time in many years.'

But role models do not have to be famous people: our friends and colleagues can help out here. My mate Maud Cook has given me the confidence to grow old gracefully and disgracefully. Now in her seventies, she is a magnificent inspiration. Maud is in the living world: she believes she is never too old to learn – and learn she does!

She started a university course when she retired. She cut her beautiful, shoulder-length hair into a quarter-inch urchin because she felt like a change of image. She reads self-development and therapy books, she writes essays, she plays cards (too well for my liking) and she paints her nails. She is actively involved in politics. She works as a volunteer with children with learning difficulties. Maud is, in sum, living proof that you don't have to be thinner than your natural weight and younger than twenty-eight to be an OK woman and lead a very successful life.

Look around and see who is making the most of their lives, and then see what you can learn from them. Watch, emulate, listen, ask direct questions and do anything else that strikes you as appropriate and helpful.

Getting started

In the returned DB questionnaires, personal development was acknowledged as a significant help in enabling women to break the diet cycle.

Personal development means stretching and developing ourselves so that we acquire:

- new skills
- new sets of feelings
- new ways of seeing things
- new attitudes
- new levels of consciousness
- new ways of managing ourselves and our affairs

In short, personal development means a different state of being or functioning.

Everything in our lives influences us, and sometimes it is not until years later that we realize what impact a particular experience has had on us. Looking back, I can identify many people, events and experiences that helped me develop and grow to the stage where I could break free. Many of them are not directly related to dieting, but their cumulative effect has been to help me develop a greater sense of self-worth and of who I am. Many routes to personal development were mentioned by the women who responded to our questionnaire. Here is a selection:

Josie: popular psychology and positive thinking books. Also, seeing a gestalt therapist has helped me regain my confidence and rely on my own judgements.

Suki: Belonging to organizations like Diet Breakers.

Polly: Therapy helped me put my feelings about size into perspective.

Diana: My therapist helped by emphasizing emotional nourishment.

Juliette: A self-help group was an enormous help in learning how to eat properly, to trust my body, to treat myself well, to live for today, not to put everything off until I was size 10 and bustless. The group gave me the courage to start swimming again.

Kay: The women's movement and consciousness-raising groups. Anti-oppressive and anti-discriminatory emphasis on a recent Diploma in Social Work course helped to sharpen my awareness, and I now see women refusing to succumb to the demands of others and proclaiming the right to be themselves.

Lorna: Diet Breakers and *DB* magazine has helped me see that this issue is not just personal – it's political, too – and how the two are interwoven.

Books and magazines were also mentioned (see Further Reading on pages 245 and 246). Many women talked about the benefits and feeling of empowerment from learning new things, linking with different women to develop new ideas, and gaining a sense of achievement in passing on their newly acquired knowledge and skills to others.

The benefits and disbenefits from your dieting behaviour

We do things for reasons which, although not always clear, are entirely legitimate for us. It may help to start by acknowledging how important dieting has been for you, and what it has provided for you – in other words, your personal pay-offs. From the list below, tick off those that you recognize in yourself, and add others to your list as they occur to you.

• It's a known entity, therefore safe and secure

- It takes my mind off other problems
- It helps me cope
- It gives me an identity
- It's second nature – I can do it without thinking too much
- I feel I'm a member of the women's club – I have a sense of belonging
- I feel in control
- I don't challenge other people and I fit in with the crowd, which makes life easy
- My behaviour makes other people feel comfortable

So this is your 'status quo' position. You are recognizing the role that dieting has played for you. Perhaps you are starting to feel angry, hurt or let down, but try not to blame yourself. At some level dieting has worked for you – albeit at a price.

Acknowledging what dieting has cost you, personally, may also be useful. Again add to the list if you want to:

- Feeling cut off
- Feeling a failure when it doesn't work
- Regrets about missing out on things/life passing me by
- I'm obsessed
- Always feeling dissatisfied with my body
- Feeling inadequate and that my confidence is sapped
- Contradictory feelings of being in and out of control
- I never feel I've achieved anything
- I don't take risks, so I don't fulfil my potential
- I've become secretive
- I feel I have nothing new to learn/I'm not open to new ideas
- I've wasted my money
- I'm on a roundabout that never actually gets anywhere
- I have no freedom to be myself

These are the costs that you have been living with but may not have considered before or revealed to those around you. There's a strong likelihood that you will feel sadness and regret, or anger and indignation, which seem to me appropriate responses when we look at this list. Dieting is a pernicious occupation.

Like the woman who knew she didn't want her daughter ending

up like her, lots of dieters have identified the negative effects of
their behaviour on others:

- My children are picking up the habit
- I irritate my partner because of my inflexibility around eating
  and eating out
- I'm not putting out to others, so I tend to be dismissed/
  isolated
- I'm taken for granted
- Some people find me boring because of my preoccupation
- I'm too intense and preoccupied in my choice of food
- I'm no pleasure to share a meal with

Can you identify with any of these? Can you think of other negative
effects that your dieting has had?

Feeling fat

For so many of us our feelings of self-esteem are measured by
our bodies, and our bodies are measured by the tape measure,
the scales and the food we've eaten. As a result our feelings get
jumbled up. We become confused about what we are really feeling,
and it all comes out as 'feeling fat'. Do you feel fat even when
you haven't been over-eating, and regardless of compliments from
others? Do you have that megaphone inside your head constantly
berating you for your inability to restrict your food intake: 'What
a pig! I've just gobbled down all that food, and now I feel really
bloated – what an idiot!' We have been encouraged to lump all
our nasty feelings into just one feeling: *fat* – and, hey presto, the
cure for this is to diet.

Although 'fat' isn't a feeling, just about every woman knows
that 'feeling fat' feeling. It is a state of mind unrelated to our
actual body size – a woman suffering from anorexia, for instance,
will tell you she feels fat. It is very important to see how this
message of fat becomes imprinted in our thoughts, so that we
all feel dissatisfied with our own bodies and fear and hate fatter
bodies even more. Thinking about these issues, appreciating the
role that dieting has played and the costs it has exacted, will

help you to put diets into perspective and reinforce your desire
to change.

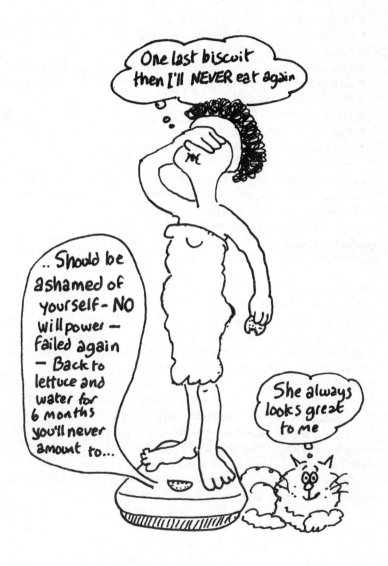

When you are 'feeling fat', try instead gently unravelling what's
behind it. Are you feeling:

- Guilty about the food you have just eaten?
- Not attractive enough?
- Put down in some way?
- Frightened?
- Bad day about work?
- Angry?
- Lonely?
- Reminded of a previous unhappy experience?
- In need of a cuddle?
- Hungry?
- Fed up or bored?
- In need of excitement?

Instead of restricting what you are eating, punishing yourself or turning to food for comfort, try to look for other ways to meet your emotional needs. Put your feelings in their proper place: if you were put down by a remark from a colleague at work, it's far better to express your feelings of hurt or anger appropriately with the person. Give yourself permission not to have to be perfect, and permission to feel. It is natural to have all these feelings and more.

Too many women walk around in fear of being found out – frightened that what we are feeling is not natural, and that if people knew what we were really like they would not like us. It isn't true. Not everybody wants Miss Goody Two Shoes for a friend. Usually they get a whiff of insincerity when our mask slips and the nasty bits start dribbling out when we least expect them. In my experience, the more I allow myself to be myself, the more I like myself, the more I meet my needs, and the more other people like me. It is true that some people shy away from me. Over the years I have found that this is because we have little in common or – I have to admit the possibility – they simply do not like me. There is a verse used in gestalt therapy that is worth keeping in mind on such occasions:

> *I am I*
> *And you are you*
> *And if we should meet*
> *It will be wonderful*
> *And if not, so be it*

I am still working on it. Give it a try for yourself and see. Only by recognizing your true feelings will you be able to set about dealing with them compassionately and appropriately. Try to accept that from childhood you have absorbed the messages that thin is good and fat is bad, and that you probably had no choice in the matter. Turn the conversation in your head to a friendlier station, such as:

- All things pass, including negative thinking about myself – so think positive.
- I am beginning to realize that I feel fat after I have eaten so-called forbidden foods which have broken my diet, or when I have binged.
- I know I turn to food for comfort, and I am getting in touch with my true feelings.
- I am stopping blaming myself for my behaviour, because I deserve more understanding and compassion.
- I realize I needed to eat that second helping of food even though I wasn't hungry. I know I am hungry for other things in my life, and I am finding out what they are so that I can feed my real need.

Since you've read this far, you probably know you want something more for yourself and are preparing yourself for change so as to be ready to move on.

The process of diet breaking

Swimming into uncharted waters, leaving a safe place for an unknown one, can be scary. We worry that we may fail and be left stranded in no-man's land with our foundations swept from under us. We are going to be different, a 'new' person in the literal sense. Will others know and recognize us? Will they like us? Will we know and recognize ourselves? Will we like ourselves? But you've come this far, and you want to do it. There are identifiable and predictable stages in the process of diet breaking. Being aware of them, and of where you are in

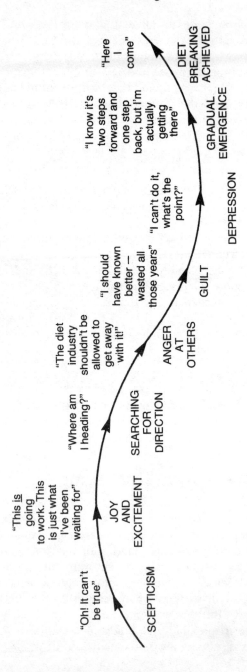

"Oh! It can't be true"

SCEPTICISM

"This is going to work. This is just what I've been waiting for"

JOY AND EXCITEMENT

"Where am I heading?"

SEARCHING FOR DIRECTION

"The diet industry shouldn't be allowed to get away with it!"

ANGER AT OTHERS

"I should have known better — wasted all those years"

GUILT

"I can't do it, what's the point?"

DEPRESSION

"I know it's two steps forward and one step back, but I'm actually getting there"

GRADUAL EMERGENCE

"Here I come"

DIET BREAKING ACHIEVED

the process, can help you identify your feelings and manage the process successfully.

We can see the steps we need to take and the barriers to overcome, but unless we understand what we are feeling we won't be able to anticipate problem areas or prevent premature failure. Typically we will feel the emotions shown in the drawing.

As dieters, when things are not going well we make the mistake of constantly going back to the starting blocks. Instead, notice where you are in the process – especially when you are not feeling good or are having second thoughts. Instead of going back to the beginning, stay where you are and work with your feelings from this position. This is not the Grand National, so give yourself time. Then, when you feel ready, move on.

Getting your support systems organized

Having people around us whom we can turn to for help and companionship is important. Generally speaking, people like to help; but for a variety of reasons they do not know how to, and so we have to tell them. Other people think they are helping but in fact are not – we have to tell them too, but more on that later. For the moment let's concentrate on getting our support systems organized.

Think for a moment about your circle of friends and family and the various things you get from them, and how each one sees and knows a different side of you. Your daughter, for example, may see the nurturing side of you, your best friend sees the playful giggler, while your colleagues see the serious businesswoman. At different times, according to the situation, you may turn to different members of your circle for support. Think about which members of your circle will provide you with support now, and in what form that support can be. Catherine wrote: 'I have a few close friends who never advise, but are always there to say the right thing when I'm down. They trust me to learn from my own mistakes, and they give me the confidence to learn and start to trust myself. They stand by me whatever I do, and help me to love and accept myself.'

We all have the ability to choose who we spend time with. Connie said: 'I make a point of being with people who don't comment constantly on my appearance, who acknowledge my feelings and help me feel good about myself generally.' Diane, who is a lesbian, has friends who find large people attractive. She finds mixing with lesbian women, who are more comfortable with their bodies, has helped her. And Lorraine wrote: 'My husband has been my greatest confidence-booster. He encourages me to look for clothes that make me look attractive at the size I am, rather than trying to lose weight to fit the fashion.'

Are your friends being as supportive as you would like? If not, ask yourself if they know what you are feeling. Penny wrote, 'Being open to my friends about my eating problem really made a difference. Before I did that they had no idea what I was going through.' Perhaps *your* friends and loved ones don't know what you are going through. It might take some courage on your part to tell them, but without taking that risk of opening up you can't really expect them to be able to offer you the love and support you need.

Unfortunately, not everyone around you will welcome you branching out and developing yourself. Some may feel threatened or inconvenienced that you want to attend a weekly group or to spend money on yourself. They may, at some level, realize that if you change they will be affected, which means they will need to change too. Perhaps you won't be around at six o'clock to cook dinner every Tuesday evening, perhaps you will prefer to spend your money on a residential workshop than on new curtains. You yourself won't know what changes there will be until the time comes – which can be both scary and exciting.

Sometimes our relationships just drift along out of habit, and no longer nourish us. And sometimes people close to us can be very unhelpful. Pat wrote, 'I always felt my ex-husband had taken me on to do me a favour. He never told me I was beautiful. He claimed that our kids got their good looks from his side of the family.' Dawn said, 'My husband hinders by belittling me. I seem to have spent twenty-five years trying to make him proud of me.' It may be painful to concede that our family and friends are impeding our progress in breaking the diet cycle. Some women recognized that distancing themselves from their loved one helped. Sophie wrote: 'I went to work abroad, and the break from family and old friends helped me. I learned to peel away lots of the old ideas, and turned those painful and embarrassing experiences into learning ones.'

If you feel your friends are not helpful, or indeed may be making things worse, it might be time to think about what these friends really offer you. Perhaps they have their own problems in connection with body-image and self-esteem, or a vested interest in keeping you hooked. Rosemary wrote, 'I had a boyfriend who constantly told me I was beautiful but that if I lost a stone I'd be even better. He also wished in my presence that he could have a Japanese girlfriend with a "neat little bottom". I'll leave it to you to decide which two parts of his anatomy were neat and little: . . . one was his brain.'

If any of this sounds familiar to you, ask yourself why you stay in a relationship that hurts you. What part are you playing in perpetuating this bind? Is it time for you to challenge what's going on? Or maybe you should even consider moving on and making way for new people to come into your life. In a long-term relationship that you are committed to, learning to challenge unhelpful behaviour in a constructive way and insisting on specific changes to your partner's behaviour will increase your feelings of empowerment. You might find some of the techniques suggested in Chapter 8 helpful. Jane says she is clear where she stands with her friends: 'Any body criticism from either friends or partner, and they get dumped. You can choose friends and boyfriends – you don't have to take crap from these two groups. Although I must admit it did take me a while to build up confidence to take this stand.'

Look at the matrix diagram on page 88 and identify people who provide the support you need. You may find that the same person provides support for you at each point on the grid – in which case, great – but if that relationship broke down or the person went away you would lose all your support in one go. Obviously the more people you can identify at each point, the better. This exercise may also help you 'discover' those you had not appreciated could be your supports. Don't forget that children and even pets can be very good supports. If you find gaps on the grid, don't despair: use it as a guide to thinking about your circle of friends and as an aid in developing relationships with people who will provide support in these particular areas for you. Your supports are really important – don't take them for granted. Think of ways in which you can support them, and let them know they are important or special to you.

Diet Breaking

Someone......

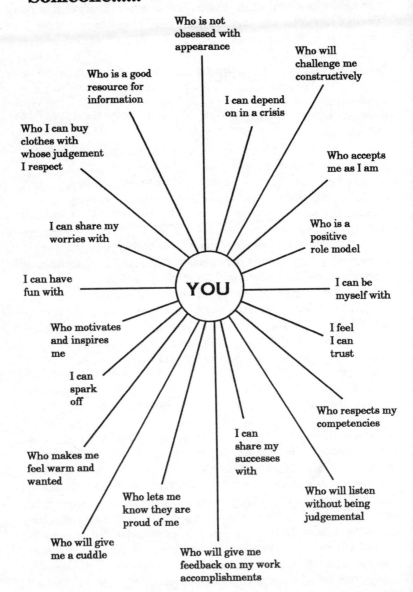

Who is not
obsessed with
appearance

Who will
challenge me
constructively

Who is a good
resource for
information

I can depend
on in a crisis

Who I can buy
clothes with
whose judgement
I respect

Who accepts
me as I am

I can share my
worries with

Who is a
positive
role model

I can have
fun with

YOU

I can be
myself with

Who motivates
and inspires
me

I feel
I can
trust

I can
spark
off

Who respects my
competencies

Who makes me
feel warm and
wanted

I can
share my
successes
with

Who will listen
without being
judgemental

Who lets me
know they are
proud of me

Who will give
me a cuddle

Who will give me
feedback on my work
accomplishments

Diet Breakers' Support Matrix

When you have worked your way round the matrix, set it aside
and come back to it later. You may have overlooked one or two
obvious supports, but these can be added at any time.

Overcoming barriers

Below is a list of reasons that women give which make it difficult
for them to stop dieting. Can you identify yourself in any of the
following statements? Again, add to the list if you wish.

- It's too hard to stop dieting – it has become a habit
- I'm frightened what might happen
- I don't want to give up hope that one day I'll be thinner
- It's not worth the effort
- I don't like to admit I got it wrong for so long
- I'm afraid to try something different
- All my friends diet – they won't understand
- My partner won't like/accept it
- If I don't diet I fear I will lose control
- People won't like me any more
- My partner might leave me
- I am worried what might happen to my looks
- My mum/sister will think I am criticizing her because she
  diets
- I like to be more attractive than other women
- My weight will balloon
- It's my hobby
- I won't know what to eat
- Dieting helps me ignore other problems
- I'll have no other excuse for . . .

Some of these barriers may be real, while others we will have
erected ourselves. When we are in the diet mentality, the positive
outcomes from stopping dieting don't get a look in. Some could
be there as excuses for our inactivity.

As you look through this list, and perhaps add to it, you will
probably find that some are more significant for you than others.
Some may not apply at all and so, naturally, you will not want

to spend time on them. Just move to the ones that are important for you.

Look at each statement carefully and ask yourself if it is relevant to you. If so, is it a real threat or does it exist only in your imagination? Think about where the fear originates. Once you can get back to the origins of the message you may be able to put the threat into perspective and find a way to deal with it. If, for example, you are afraid what might happen if you stop dieting, you could try talking to your partner, parents, relatives or friends about wanting to stop dieting and your fears – you may be pleasantly surprised. If you believe your weight will balloon you may need to reread Chapter 3 or seek more information on the realities and failures of diets (see Further Reading).

Each barrier will have a different fear level. Rank them in order from moderately feared to most feared. Start by tackling the least feared ones, and enjoy the feeling of success as you overcome them. This way you won't be setting yourself up for early failure, and will be building confidence to deal with your more feared barriers later on. What I have discovered is that, having confronted the least feared barriers, the most feared ones don't seem so bad and sometimes just fizzle away.

Let's take as a working example the fear that your mum will feel criticized when you stop dieting. Confronting our parents can in itself be liberating. It represents an important step in our journey of emancipation, because we are beginning to define and set our own rules rather than following Mum and Dad. Nevertheless many of us find such a confrontation difficult, so to avoid unnecessary tears try to think things through a little first. If your mother has been dieting for the last thirty years, it is very likely that she will see your decision to stop as a threat or criticism – to her standards and values, her way of life, her abilities as a mother, her attractiveness, her womanhood even. So your fears may be justified, but you may still feel you need to talk to her about your decision to stop dieting. If this is the case, prepare yourself and do your best to pick a good time; some of the techniques suggested in Chapter 7 may help you. And remember, you are now making decisions that are best for you – not for your mum. So although she may be unhappy or angry, you can still be right! Finally, if you don't live with your mother, do you actually need to tell her about your decision to ditch dieting?

Self-affirmations

Our thoughts affect our feelings, which impact on our behaviour. The thoughts/conversations we have with ourselves are very important. Many dieters' self-talk is more like a personal megaphone, ever ready to berate us. Changing our self-talk into statements which affirm our personalities and positive qualities helps to promote positive thoughts about ourselves, which in turn can help us feel more confident. Affirmations should be made in the present tense, and not be too long. Lists of ideas for affirmations are given below, and you can add others of your own. When I first started working with affirmations, I was staggered to hear the suggestion that we say our positive affirmations at least two hundred times a day. But when I think how often our negative megaphone pipes up, perhaps it wasn't an over-prescription.

I believe that any positive affirmations are good. Saying them when you feel good is obviously easiest, and the more you say them the easier it gets – although it can still feel embarrassing. I find affirmations helpful to counter 'everyday' negative self-talk, but not helpful or realistic when I am feeling awful or have a real problem. I prefer to try to deal with the issue of the moment, and then go back to the affirmations.

When your negative self-talk is very destructive it helps to challenge it, so this first list includes a number of challenges.

- It is dieting that cuts me off
- It is diets that have failed, not me
- It is not too late to stop dieting
- I am beginning to release my obsession
- My body serves me well
- I am working to feel stronger and more confident
- As I break the diet cycle I have more confidence
- I achieve a lot and am having success in starting to break with dieting
- I choose when to take risks
- I am willing to learn and am open to new ideas

Take notice of what you are actually saying to yourself that is damaging. But do so slowly – our thoughts come so fast sometimes that we can miss something vital. You may find it helpful to write

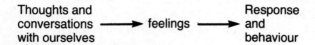

Constantly looking for faults, pecking away at ourselves, erodes our self esteem. It is a vicious circle.

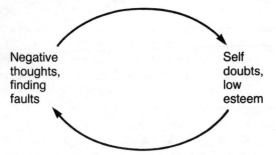

Changing negative thoughts and self talk helps build our confidence.

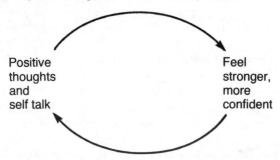

it down. When you have done this, come up with a challenge to the negative self-talk and write that down too. Give yourself time, and then come up with a positive message for yourself and write that down. You may find it helpful to write your positive message on a Post-it and stick it on the bathroom mirror, or write it in your diary – anywhere you can see and read it often.

Here is a list of general affirmations. Again, just use this list as a guide, and to try to write ones that suit you personally. Write your affirmations out and stick them around your home. Carry them with you, as well, to use as little 'pep-ups' whenever the old megaphone starts droning on.

- I have the desire to break the habit
- I am worth the effort
- I am breaking free
- By taking one step at a time I am making it easier for myself
- I ask for support from others
- I forgive myself if I have setbacks – and will move on

Helping or hindering?

There will undoubtedly be some unhelpful people or influences around you, so we must somehow reduce the degree to which they hinder your progress. Constantly weighing yourself will not help you. Weighing scales do not measure the goals you are aiming for, nor do tape measures. Using these items when you have a difficulty or a bad day can lead you back into the diet trap and divert you from dealing with your problem.

Clothes that do not fit you merely chastise you and stop you from accepting yourself right now and from living in the present. Hanging on to any clothes that do not fit you – whether they are too large or too small – prevents you from accepting yourself as you are now. After diet breaking for a while you may discover that your body returns to its natural weight. If this is lower than you have been of late, throw out or have altered any clothes that are too big for you. But if you have not lost weight, please don't regard your diet breaking as a failure too. We are not all meant to be thin. Remind yourself that your aim was not to get thinner – it was to be healthier and happier.

Magazines that promote a thin-is-best message, or where all the features and adverts show very young women, are also hindrances because they are perpetuating the tyranny. We are not all young, we are not all thin, we are not all white and we don't want to be sidetracked or ignored. So surround yourself with positive images and influences that are more in tune with the diet breaking approach.

Look at the people in your life and make sure you spend time with those who boost your confidence and who make you feel good when you are with them. Go out of your way to develop relationships with people who project a positive image themselves and who want more from life than just another diet. Reduce the amount of time you spend with people who try to bring you down or get in the way of your progress. They have their own agenda – leave them to work their way through it.

Reality check

Very few things in life go completely smoothly and according to plan – including diet breaking. There are always some days that are better than others. You must expect that. So avoid unrealistic expectations – and then you won't be nearly as disappointed. Nobody is 100 per cent perfect and unable to make a mistake. Go easy on yourself, allow yourself to be human. Approach each day and each step as a progression on your journey. You are not playing Monopoly and there are no penalties or fines: after a setback or a bad day you don't have to go to jail or back to base. Just carry on from where you are.

Pacing yourself

Resist an all-or-nothing approach – you're not going for a target weight or trying to reduce two dress sizes in three weeks. You are developing a range of goals, short- and long-term, that are enriching, achievable and sustainable. They are personal to you, not imposed from a diet sheet, a television ad or the next door neighbour. Nor, on the other hand, should you procrastinate.

There needs to be an element of challenge and of you stretching yourself to move forward.

Keeping a journal

I find it very helpful to keep a journal. I use it to write down my thoughts and feelings and to register my successes. I record my dreams sometimes, too, and write down affirmations. When I read back I can sometimes make sense of a particular feeling or event, or make connections, or see a pattern to my behaviour. And when there is no one around to talk to about my feelings, writing things down helps too. I have been keeping my journal for eight years, and it is very pleasurable to see how I have grown in some areas. Some things have changed; others haven't changed, but my feelings about them have; and then there are some things I am still dealing with. If you haven't tried keeping a journal, you might like to give it a try. But don't get bogged down into feeling you *must* write in your journal. Write when you feel like it. Keep it in a safe place, and make it clear to those you live with that it is private.

Rewarding yourself

Enjoy your journey and validate your successes as they happen. Measure your achievements yourself, and don't let others take them away from you. Find ways to reward yourself. The thinking goes something like: this step is a bit challenging, I'm going to have a go at it, and my reward will be a bunch of flowers, or a walk in the park, or a nice long bath. You will feel good about an achievement, and a reward is a concrete recognition of your effort. A note or tick in your journal against a barrier that you have overcome is a reward in itself.

Because we have been dieting for so long, the thought of not dieting can be very scary. Many women fear they will over-eat if they are not dieting. Because we have been regulating our food intake unnaturally (through dieting), we need to learn to start trusting ourselves again.

In my experience, over-eating comes from deprivation. It could be deprivation of food, emotional support or some other need. If you have been working on the suggestions in this chapter you will be starting to feel stronger about your own abilities and beginning to meet your emotional needs in more appropriate ways.

The fear of over-eating, or all-or-nothing eating, is symptomatic of the diet mentality:

- If I don't diet, I over-eat
- If I start to eat, I eat it all

The opposite of dieting is not over-eating. The opposite of dieting is eating, enjoying food and putting diets in their proper place – in the bin!

Pauline is on her way . . .

Like many women I have been conned into believing that to be slim will give me everything, and therefore have been on a constant diet all my life from the age of about fifteen. I am now thirty-eight.

I could tell you every calorie in almost every food as I've made it my lifetime's obsession, but the ironic thing is that my preoccupation with food has made me grow larger, as I eat to compensate for things in life. However, I've decided I want to jump off the merry-go-round, eat healthily, exercise and relax about the whole subject.

I expect you will hear from many more ladies like myself. It's so lovely to hear the other side of the coin, that there is life after THE DIET. Thank you so much. Diet Breakers has helped me as an individual to get everything into perspective – as women we can love ourselves for just being ourselves, with all our spiritual and creative gifts.

5

What to Eat and Enjoy Now You Don't Diet

I don't believe it!

So what can you eat and enjoy now you don't diet? Answer: *anything*!

Yes, you did read it correctly: you can eat anything you want. There's no con. No ifs and buts. No magic formula about how you eat and when you eat. No one day on and one day off. I am not saying you can eat anything you want so long as:

- you stand up when you're eating
- you chew each bite 189 times
- you eat it from a small bowl
- it has less than 15 calories
- you eat half a grapefruit first
- you mix proteins and carbohydrates
- it doesn't have a 'z' in its name
- you've had a blood test first
- it's a Monday, Wednesday or Friday
- you don't swallow it
- the month has more than thirty-one days
- you don't like the taste of it
- it doesn't answer you back

OK – so I stretched the list of new/magic/special diets a little, but you get my drift. Perhaps you recognize one or two from some regime you have tried in the past.

Dieters are regularly introduced to new and wondrous methods of eating or formulae that outsmart our bodies, our food, our taste buds and our common sense. Of course they don't work in terms of weight loss, but they may provide us with more misplaced hope. Unfortunately the hopes swiftly turn to disappointment when we have not stuck to the mandatory eight boiled eggs a day.

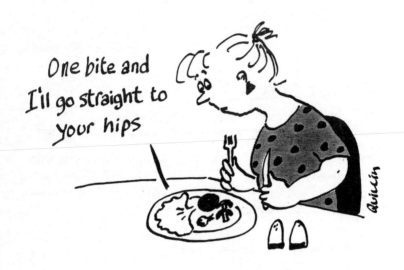

A couple of years back I read in the newspapers about the ice cream diet, guaranteed to help you lose 8 pounds a week. All you had to do was eat a tub of ice cream after breakfast and another after lunch, and two tubs after dinner in the evening. Apparently it swept through a number of towns in the north-east of England, and hundreds of people tried the diet. Helpful folk passed the diet sheet on to their friends. Many thought it seemed too good to be true, yet, throwing away all their common sense, still had a go: they gave it a week and noticed the difference.

Many reported being absolutely sick of ice cream. One woman had developed a red rash on her face and upper body. Others just found the diet had not worked – they had not lost weight. A number had actually put on weight.

We can become so desperate to find a diet we can stick to that we will literally believe anything. Yet, even if they did work, in the long run such gimmicks are not good for us because they alienate us from food and the pleasure of eating naturally for energy. As a result of the diet mentality, childhood conditioning or misleading information put out by the slimming and advertising industries too many people have become confused about food and have developed a fear of it.

Which is why you may have balked at my suggestion that you can eat anything. Just remember that there is no such thing as good and bad food. Food is food is food. It is meant to be eaten and enjoyed, not feared or forbidden.

Rediscover your natural abilities

We all possess the abilities to find answers to our problems with food and dieting. With a bit of gentle coaxing and practice you can rekindle your natural skills to choose the right food for you. To a woman gripped in the diet mentality this may seem hard to swallow in one go, so let's take it a step at a time.

Dr Marion Hetherington is a psychologist at Dundee University who specializes in eating and eating disorders. Marion dedicates much of her time to watching people eat, and finds that women are not as willing as men to take part in experimental studies which involve foods that they regard as forbidden – even if they like these foods. Indeed, many decline the very foods that are, by their own ratings, the most pleasant.

Many women feel guilty about eating foods they enjoy, and punish themselves for not resisting them. Sometimes they salve the guilt by eating secretly. However, eating secretly doesn't really help, because deep down you know what you've eaten. It helps, I believe, to stop regarding foods as good or bad, safe or forbidden.

There is plenty of evidence to support the claim that diet and nutrition are very important to good health; we all know that. But in recent years another form of food guilt-tripping has developed with the notion of healthy and unhealthy foods, which serves to mask or even to encourage faddy eating. I am talking about such things as raw vegetable and fruit diets or the so-called low toxin or 'combining' diets.

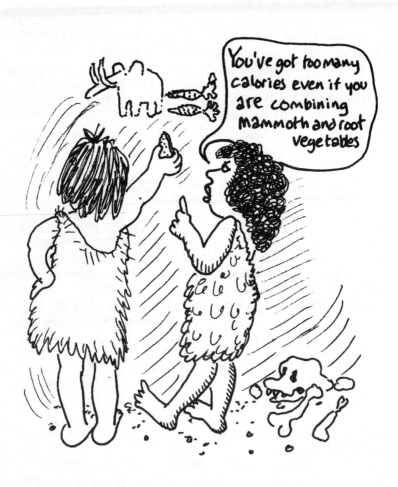

We could be forgiven for forgetting that human beings have survived for millions of years without counting calories or worrying too much about expelling the toxins from their bodies or eating only raw vegetables. How ever did our ancestors manage?

The conditioning process: what we teach children

So, where do we learn what to eat? How do we discover what food we like and enjoy? Where do we get the idea that some foods are good and bad? And who teaches us to diet?

In all societies, adults teach their children eating and table manners. It's a long, slow process, because we are being taught not only what and how to eat, but also the value system of the society or group into which we have been born.

Before young children start learning the emotional overtones that may be attached to food, they are quite capable of selecting a nutritious, well-balanced diet. At just a few months old babies know what they like and it is a joy to watch them taste and savour various foods, enthusiastically demanding more of the things they like and unceremoniously spitting out what they don't want.

Unfortunately, by the time we are two or three years old our parents may unwittingly have started our training in the diet mentality. We will already have started associating different emotions and values and identities with various foods, and these associations can stay with us for the rest of our lives.

Some of the messages we picked up may seem useful and sensible training for children. For example, who wasn't told to eat their greens? Or that crusts will make your teeth and gums strong? And you had to finish your main course before you could have any pudding. However, studies show that attempting to coerce and cajole children to eat certain foods and to reject others does not work. In fact it has the opposite effect to the one our parents intended.

Did you, for example, eat and enjoy crusts more in the knowledge that they would make your teeth and gums stronger? No, neither did I. Nor did I like my spinach and cabbage better. On the other hand chips, trifle, apple pie, chocolates and sweets still tasted just as delicious with the knowledge that they were rotting my teeth or were bad in some other way, and so the seeds of guilt were planted.

Over the years those seeds were nurtured, watered and delivered to me through a variety of messengers: my parents and family, friends, the school dinner lady who made me sit in the dining hall eating lamb stew and pearl barley until I gagged, the wider community, the advertising and diet industries who talk of 'no need to feel guilty', and well-meaning health professionals. I was taught – and I bet you were, too – to eat certain foods and cut back or cut out others. I heard what they said. I understood every word. But they did not motivate me.

In fact the very things I was told to cut back on became, by definition, more enticing and appealing. Such a clever line in that ad for cream cakes: 'naughty but nice'. When was the last time you longed for cabbage, cottage cheese, crusts and lettuce leaves?

Indeed, parental messages such as eating our greens don't just encourage a child's natural sense of rebellionsness but also, like diet products, help to inculcate children with the diet mentality. What they do is lead the young to disregard their internal physiological cues for regulating their intake, and encourage them to rely on external ones.

Perhaps our desire to control children's eating stems from an assumption that they cannot control their own food intake. This probably comes from the fact that for years we adults have felt unable to control our own eating, so we believe our internal hunger cues are at best unreliable but, more likely, faulty or non-existent. That could be why you have difficulty accepting the fact that you can eat anything you want: for a very long time you have received messages that you can't be trusted because what you want is wrong, bad, dangerous, naughty, and that if you have what you want you will go out of control. If you have been subsisting on foods which you find unexciting, it is hardly surprising that when you react against this restrictive regime you'll head straight for the tasty foods, usually high in fat and calories. This has been borne out in preliminary studies at Yale University, in which women yo-yo dieters have shown a greater preference for dietary fat than they did before they began dieting.

And if you think that's the only downside to yo-yo dieting, take a look at this list of effects given by Tom Sanders and Peter Bazalgette:

- decreases in lean tissue (including heart muscle)
- loss of bone minerals
- attacks of gout or gallstones
- cardiac arrhythmias, leading to sudden heart attacks
- hair loss

- fibrosis and scarring of tissue
- refeeding hypertension (high blood pressure when returning to a normal diet)
- depression
- harmful side-effects of appetite-depressant drugs
- shortened lifespan

The bad-feelings-and-eating-for-comfort cycle

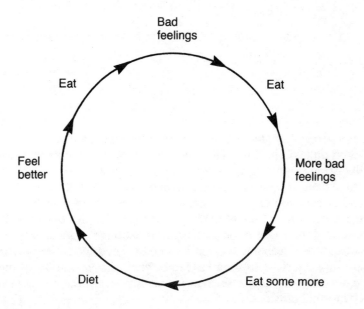

Chocolate is a popular comforter. (Apart from tasting absolutely delicious, it can also give us a buzz because it contains a mood-lifting chemical called beta phenylethylamine and refined carbohydrates for a boost of instant energy.

When we eat chocolate and sweets, the body reacts by pumping out insulin to bring our blood sugar level down. If it drops lower

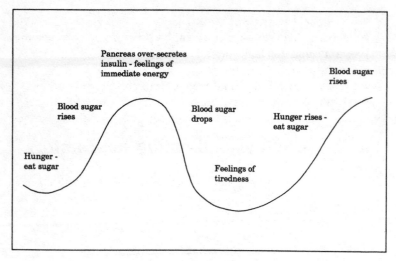

Blood Sugar Roller Coaster

than before you ate the chocolate, you then want another bar, and so on and so on. So eating sweet things on an empty stomach is like taking our body for a ride on a roller coaster.

By being aware of how the human body reacts to chocolates and sweets you can make informed choices about what you eat and when you eat it – not on an empty stomach, for example. Be aware of the psychological aspect, too. Turning to food for some comfort is reasonable enough – after all, good food is very nice. However, turning to food instead of getting your real needs met is not so good – because food is unlikely to have any long-term comforting effect.

Getting to know hunger again

Do you know what it feels like to be hungry? I didn't know what it felt like for going on twenty years. For me, eating had nothing to do with hunger. It had to do with seeing food and wanting it. It also had to do with fear – fear of not getting enough, of being with

other people, of not being good enough, of not feeling confident
. . . and fear of being hungry.

When I started to allow myself to feel hungry I realized it isn't so
frightening after all. For me, it feels like butterflies in my stomach
which turn to rumblings, and then I feel light-headed and faint if
I don't feed myself. Now that I know what it feels like it doesn't
frighten me any more, and I feed myself when I get the familiar
butterflies. By being more in touch with how it feels to be hungry,
and only then eating, I am better able to notice when I have had
enough to eat.

Nowadays I often have a drink instead of eating, because I have
found that I may be thirsty rather than hungry. Before, I did not
realize – I was not able to differentiate between hunger and thirst
until I was famished.

Why don't you try this technique? Experience how your body
feels when it's hungry – and then feed it.

I have also found that the more often I respond appropriately to
my physical hunger, the better I am able to deal with my emotional
needs. I don't have so many mood swings, I don't feel so tired, and
I don't beat myself with feelings of guilt the way I used to. Don't
get me wrong – I am not saying I never get cross or angry, or that I
never feel fed up. What I am saying is that, when I do feel this way,
it is not because of food and dieting; since I stopped my twenty-plus
years of full-time dieting I don't get nearly so many bad moments;
and because the dieting is not blurring the issues I can more easily
work out what is wrong.

Dealing with snacking and nibbling

When asked what external cues trigger off eating, women frequently identify the following:

- Feeling: bored, worried, angry, unhappy, frustrated
- Lifestyle: watching television or reading magazines, especially
  ones featuring food or diets
- Seeing: other people eating enticing foods, advertisements,
  food in shop windows
- Hearing: the crackle of crisps, someone biting an apple,
  people talking about delicious food

- Thinking: about the piece of cake, the Mars bar, the ice cream in the freezer
- Smelling: freshly brewed coffee, hot bread, fish and chips, frying bacon, doughnuts, curry
- Tasting: the first bite of the nicest . . . must have more peanuts, chips, etc.

They tell me that they pick up the cue to eat something, fancy it, eat it (whether they are hungry or not), and then feel unhappy or guilty. Usually these foods are tempting tit-bits or snacks, such as peanuts or crisps. At parties I have known myself to eat a bowl of peanuts and then go looking for more – before the food is served.

What I do now is give myself a bit of time before eating whatever it is I fancy. Because I don't allow myself to become ravenously hungry, I don't confuse external and internal cues. So I give myself a bit of time, and perhaps have a drink. Then, ten or fifteen minutes later, if I still want it I have it. Often I don't want it. But if I do, I enjoy it.

Where possible I put snacks on a plate rather than nibbling from a bag. Nibbling sounds insignificant – until you realize you've nibbled your way through a large bag of crisps. So, on to the plate they go. I can see what they look like and how many there are, eat them, enjoy and savour them, and then stop when I've had enough.

The reconditioning process: let's learn from children

Contrary to our insecurities, studies have shown that children who are left to their own devices – that is, who are not controlled or coerced by adults – are capable of selecting an adequate diet and, what's more, show a marked absence of feeding problems. This is what we, as diet-breaking adults, are also aiming to achieve:

- trusting ourselves to make the right choices of food for ourselves
- responding to our own internal cues
- developing a sense of self-reliance

My five-year-old grandson Alex really enjoys his food, and is very particular and enthusiastic about what he eats. He loves pasta and shepherd's pie, tuna and cucumber sandwiches, poached rather than scrambled eggs, lots of fruit, broccoli, curry, fish and chips, prawns, sweets, ice cream, rice pudding – the list is endless. When he came to stay with us for the weekend, he ate the following.

Saturday

- *Breakfast*: leftover pasta, a small bowl of porridge, half a slice of cheese on toast, five cherries, a banana, a small glass of water, half a strawberry milk shake
- *Mid-morning*: a quarter of an apple, half a glass of diluted pineapple juice
- *Lunch*: half a cheese and tomato roll, six slices of cucumber (requested on a separate plate), a quarter of an apple, a tiny bunch of grapes, a mini Mars bar, half a glass of diluted orange juice
- *Afternoon*: one slice of wholemeal bread with peanut butter and cucumber, a glass of water. Later: two cream crackers, one with cheese, the other with ham
- *Dinner*: two fresh grilled sardines, potatoes, broccoli, peas, a small piece of bread, a glass of milk

Sunday

- *Breakfast*: cornflakes and milk, half a banana, a glass of diluted orange juice, a slice of toast with peanut butter
- *Mid-morning*: half a peanut butter, cheese and tomato sandwich, a banana, a mini Milky Way, a glass of water
- *Lunch*: two rounds of baked beans on toast, a small glass of diluted pineapple juice, eight cherries (counted out by Alex)
- *Afternoon*: an eggcup full of milk, but nothing to eat
- *Dinner*: two or three crisps before dinner, then roast chicken, stuffing, one roast potato, three new potatoes, French beans, frozen peas, no gravy, followed by apple crumble and custard, and a glass of water

- Alex declined a packet of Smarties, an egg and bacon breakfast, and cheese after dinner on Sunday. He took seconds of
  broccoli and pasta

Children can be wonderfully precise, and so can we. Looking at
the list, you might think he had a lot to eat. He is a healthy, active
little boy. He needs a lot to eat, because his body needs energy to
get on with his busy life. And so does yours.

It isn't that Alex and other children have some special gift
or ability around food. We all have the ability to know when
our body needs food (although we may have lost sight of it).
A control mechanism, part of a gland called the hypothalamus
which is located at the base of our brain, tells us when we need
to eat food and also when we've had enough. In other words, it is
an internal cue. Diets, parents, calorie counting, weight watching
and so on are all external cues. We have, in effect, ignored and
over-ridden our natural abilities with food. What we need to do is
start trusting ourselves again – slowly, gently and skilfully getting
back in touch with our bodies.

I know that may sound fanciful, and perhaps you are thinking,
'I'll never be able to trust my hypothalamus.' That's what I would
have said a few years ago (had I known I'd got one). But, as the
secondhand car salesman says, trust me! Actually, don't trust me
– try it! In fact, if you did but know it, you are probably already
doing it to an extent.

Do you ever have unexpected and sudden cravings for things –
something sweet, a pickled onion, slice of toast? Surprise, surprise,
this is likely to be because your body needs a specific nutrient which
a slice of toasted cheese or whatever will provide. The more you
respond to your body, the easier it becomes.

At first this was really frightening for me. It was probably
because I had either denied myself everything or, as a lapsed
dieter, I was saying 'Oh, what the hell, go for it!' My poor little
hypothalamus was squeaking away, but all I heard was the Danish
pastry calling me from the patisserie. So I'd eat it, feel rotten and
then go back on the diet, again ignoring my hypothalamus and
thinking – constantly, longingly, lovingly – about food.

In *Fat Chance* Jane Ogden gave an example of how the
diet mentality affects our thinking around food: dieters who
were invited to participate in a taste test were given either a

'forbidden' food like chocolate, or a neutral one like a cream cracker, beforehand. The dieters given the 'forbidden' food ate more during the test than those given the neutral food. Comments like 'Now I've eaten that, I might as well make the most of it' were common.

A happy balance

We are told that we are what we eat, meaning that food is of considerable importance to our health. We can't alter the genes we were born with, but we can choose the foods we eat, and there is lots of evidence that good foods can positively aid our good health. But eating good food or a healthy diet doesn't mean you have to become a slave to some regime – the whole point of this book and of Diet Breakers is to help you liberate yourself from regimes. Nor do you have to become a faddy eater, health fanatic or culinary snob. What I am talking about is making informed choices and then eating a nutritious, well-balanced diet. And making informed choices requires only a little knowledge and common sense, not a PhD in nutrition. So relax – the Diet Breaking way of eating does not require you to become either a gourmet or a gourmand:

- A gourmet spends much of her time thinking about, planning, shopping, preparing and eating food. She enjoys being seen eating – often special delicacies that we riff-raff have never heard of.
- A gourmand enjoys eating and never misses an opportunity to do so. She always has seconds, cleans all plates and likes to leave the table feeling full up or even bloated.

Providing you are happy and healthy, there is nothing wrong with being a gourmet or a gourmand. On the other hand, if you are over-relying on food you may be compensating for something else. Perhaps something is hurting you, or is wrong, or missing from your life. By focussing on food you may be removing yourself from the here and now. Or perhaps by eating special food you are getting some form of reassurance that you are a special person. When you succeed in breaking the diet mentality and are responding to your internal hunger cues and feeling properly fed, you are, in effect, taking care of yourself in the most basic way. As you begin to take responsibility for meeting your physical hunger needs, the more secure and cared for you will feel. You will then be in a stronger position to address your emotional needs appropriately rather than turning to food. It also means you will start learning to respect food properly.

Preparing and cooking food for yourself and others can be very liberating, because it allows you to select your own ingredients and to assemble and cook them to your liking. Dr Mihaly Csikszentmihalya, Professor of Psychology at the University of Chicago and author of *Flow: The Psychology of Optimal Experience*, has shown that cooking helps create a feeling of being in control, of making things happen – like riding a bicycle, driving a car or playing a musical instrument. We are able to forget ourselves because the activity requires a certain degree of concentration. Compare this to the feelings you get when buying and eating pre-prepared meals.

- Are you able to forget yourself?
- Do you concentrate as you undo the packet?
- Do you feel in control and creative?

Or are you usually rushing home after a hard day's work, feeling a bit guilty about what you ate earlier, and wanting to balance the debt? Or knackered and keen to put your feet up and watch your favourite TV soap? If, after a heavy day, you're throwing food in the micro, eating as you watch the box, wanting to put it all behind you and feel better, cooking comes up trumps again. Perhaps surprisingly, the same study has shown that actually preparing and cooking our own food helps us to feel better than watching television. And watching television while eating means we are not actually concentrating on the food, so we miss out on the taste and pleasure and don't notice how much or how little we have eaten.

Don't despair! I am not suggesting you have to come home and prepare a gourmet meal in order to gain that feeling of creativeness and pro-activity and control. Cooking doesn't have to be an art form – preparing a nice meal does not have to be like the Last Night of the Proms.

Also, think about the times when you go shopping. Are you tired and hungry, rushing to pick up your children (who are also tired and hungry)? How about getting a little more organized, and doing a bulk shop at the weekends when you have more time? If you go shopping when you're knackered, it's no wonder you need that Kit-Kat just to give you the energy to get your purchases home.

A word about the Kit-Kat. There's nothing wrong with it. You can have one any time – although I would advise you to have it after a meal rather than before, and to eat and savour it rather than shove it in simply because you must have something – anything.

But there is something else going on here, too, because nipping into the supermarket on our way home from work is often not nipping in at all. It's struggling through the aisles, handbag over the shoulder, workbag or briefcase in left hand, basket in the other, trying to reach things at the back of the freezer and then, having managed this assault course, heading for the checkout. A chance to relax – as we queue for ten or fifteen minutes.

This is not time-saving nor relaxing nor empowering. No wonder a gin and tonic is needed as soon as you get in (let alone that Kit-Kat just to get you to the door)! But the time spent in the supermarket is conveniently left out of the equation in the adverts, isn't it? Some fresh bread, cheese and tomatoes picked up at the corner shop or deli would really save you time and money.

In these days of labour-saving devices and convenience foods, what are we spending all this new-found time on? We are spending more time on our appearance and more time watching television being told what we should be eating, how to save time and how we should look!

Registered Dietitian and author of YOU COUNT, *Calories Don't*, Linda Omichinski suggests that when you are preparing your food you aim for a quarter of your plate to contain protein-rich food and three-quarters to be carbohydrate-rich. This is a rough guide to what's healthy, and no calorie counting is required. Two-thirds, one-third is an equally good balance if you prefer it that way. Carbohydrates release energy quickly, whereas proteins release it more slowly.

Notice how you feel after each meal and how long it is between them. I know, for instance, that I need more food in the mornings. I am hungry again after three to four hours. So if I have breakfast at, say, eight, then by 11.30 or noon I am ready for lunch. In the afternoon, on the other hand, I don't want to eat much until about six o'clock. The important thing is to find what works for you, to experiment and to enjoy your food.

Try to refrain from inflicting rigid (and boring) rules on your eating such as: Monday it's shepherd's pie, Tuesday means leeks, and on Fridays we have fish and chips, or 'I always eat sandwiches for lunch.' Your nutritional needs are not static. They depend on your health at any particular time, and your circumstances – what you are doing, how relaxed you are. These all affect what your body needs at any given mealtime, so be flexible.

When you are watching TV adverts for food and diet products, try to work out their hidden message. Are you being persuaded that if you eat such and such a brand of baked beans you'll be a better mum? Or that if you eat 'Queenie's Cuisine' you'll be more sophisticated? Or modern? Or is it that the old man will just adore you more? There's usually some such message there, trying to work its way into our psyche. It's called aspirational marketing. What these ads are attempting to do is appeal to our aspirations, and sometimes they buy into our in-built snobbery too: if we eat their product we will be different, better than Them Next Door – the real or imagined slobs.

Doing it your way, for yourself

There's another kind of food snobbery which doesn't involve advertisements, but does appeal to our aspirations. That's the 'posh nosh' brigade who know where to buy Chinese lettuce leaves marinated in crab's sweat for five years, which we 'simply must have' when our friends come for brunch! Sometimes we adopt this approach to food because we need to be different from (better than) the rest, or it may provide us with a sense of belonging to the 'in crowd'. And there's nothing wrong with the 'in crowd' – or any other crowd. The point is, is it working for you?

Of course, nice food is nice food – and, for the record, I won't be turning down any invitations to Raymond Blanc's Manoir aux Quat' Saisons in Oxfordshire or Alice Waters' Chez Panise in San Francisco! I am all for nice food. What I am asking is; are you eating food *for you*? Is it what you fancy and enjoy? Or is there some other reason? Will eating this plate of porridge make you feel a lesser person than Eggs Benedict? If so, what is it that Eggs Benedict seems to give you? Ask yourself: what do you fancy to eat?

- Don't rush your food – taste it, enjoy it
- Have a rest during your meal
- Stop when you are full
- You don't have to eat it all now – you can have the rest later

There are no rules. You can have last night's dinner for breakfast, or breakfast at lunchtime – whatever you fancy, whenever you fancy it.

Of course you want to provide nice food when your friends come for a meal – but does it really have to be lobster and truffles which are hard to find and expensive? Are you trying to create an image to present to your friends? Do you need to impress them that much? (Will they in fact be impressed?) Will they really love you more? Or have they come to see you and enjoy your company? Remember, you are doing this for you – not to create a show for others. Simple food, carefully selected and prepared, is enough to do the trick. You'll feel better, save money and be healthier. Just relax, and enjoy.

Getting started

Let's now start moving towards your goal of eating what you want within the structure of a well-balanced diet – in terms of both what you eat and why you eat it. The first step is the hardest:

- Try not to use food as a reward
- You deserve nice food!
- Allow yourself to eat the foods you like and enjoy

I found that having a number of interests not related to food, and which give me stimulation, satisfaction and a feeling of control, helped me to put food where it belongs: in the cupboard, in the fridge, on the plate or in my mouth – not inside my head all day long!

- Do you have enough interests not related to food? Is there anything else you can do? Are there any interests or hobbies that you fancy trying?

- Think of two things that you are not presently doing – they do not have to be grand – that you could enjoy, would provide some stimulation, and do not cost too much money, e.g. crosswords, a pen friendship, embroidery, gardening, jigsaws, cycling, yoga, swimming.

I find that playing cards is a brilliant way to help me switch off from other things. I relax from the pressures of everyday life and am stimulated when I am playing – because I want to win.

When you get the balance right, food stops being a support or reward. So, think about how you are spending your time in terms of high stimulation activities, low stimulation ones, satisfaction and so on.

Remember to make any changes to your eating habits slowly – you don't have to do everything tonight. In fact, it is best not to try to change too many things all at once. That would put you under stress, and the changes probably would not last. And then there are the people you live with. If you were to go home tonight and declare a new way of eating you are likely to get one of two responses:

- Oh, not again!
  or
- We don't like it, we don't want it!

And so your new way of eating is likely to be sabotaged by your nearest and dearest before it's even got off the ground. But even if they didn't respond like this, remember what I said earlier: we have been learning our eating habits since we were children. Overnight changes are not likely to last, because you won't have changed your eating habits or your tastes and you will still be wanting your usual food.

We are going for small, easy steps that lead to success. Any change can be hard and stressful, which is why small steps are easier than long ones. When we are under stress it is hard to commit ourselves to – and keep – long-term goals, and this one certainly is a long-term goal. Another reason is that we Brits are proud of our traditionalist ways of doing things, and sometimes view new ideas with suspicion. Indeed, the evidence shows that the faster people make changes, the faster they give those changes up.

So we're taking the Slow Train to Georgia for a better way of living – not the Chattanooga Choo-Choo back into the shunting yard!

The problem with the the slow train route is that it takes longer. Unlike those magic diet formulas, I am not promising a difference in three days. But, unlike the magic formulas, this route works. It takes time, but you can do it. I am not saying it is easy. Of course it isn't easy. We all know that. If it were easy you would not be the veteran of many failed diets.

Are you asking yourself, 'OK, so how much weight will I lose?' If so, think again. A better question would be, 'How much happier will I be?' or 'Will I be healthier?' The answer to the last two is certainly 'Yes'. The answer to the first is 'Maybe' – but that's secondary to your health and wellbeing, surely?

- Think of all the things you can do or think about in your new-found time – the time you would have been thinking about food and dieting
- Think of the freedom to enjoy food – without feeling guilty
- Think of the healthy messages you will be passing on to your children

Perhaps there are other pay-offs for you. Think for a moment: what are the pay-offs for me in developing a healthy, balanced diet? The more pay-offs you can identify, the better – these are your motivators. Write them down somewhere – in your journal, on the wall, on a card in your handbag, anywhere that you can access easily – to remind yourself whenever you feel in need of a little boost or things are feeling tough. Don't be hard on yourself. Take each day as it comes, gently.

Are you feeling reluctant to try this new way of eating? If so, take a little time to consider what might be behind your reluctance.

- Are you scared of the prospect of not dieting?
- What scares you?
- Are you frightened you will feel out of control?
- What do you fear might happen?
- Has dieting become a habit for you?
- What could you do instead?

You may find it helpful to talk these points through with

someone who will listen. But don't ask for advice. Don't say, 'What would you do?' or 'What do you think?' We are not talking about what they would do or what they think – this is about you and what is right for you. Choose a friend who will help you think it through, consider starting a Women Against The Tyranny of Thinness group (see Chapter 9) or else go to see a trained counsellor or therapist. Remember, this is an important stage in your life that you are embarking on. Give yourself every chance to succeed.

6

Body Matters

There is much more to our bodies than simply being fashion accessories, clothes horses, advertising commodities or desirable objects. Our body is our home, where we live. We cannot trade it in for a newer, fresher, younger model. What we can do is welcome our body back, grow to love and appreciate it, and keep it in good working order.

Take a few moments to think about your body and the marvellous tasks it performs for you every day.

If you want to be proud of your body as it takes you through life, you need to keep it well maintained to give you the maximum mileage, comfort and pleasure. This means focussing both on the inside – keeping ourselves in good working order physically, emotionally and mentally, and on the outside – how we present ourselves. So in this chapter we shall be working on maintenance and in Chapter 7 we shall be looking at presentation.

The problem of stress

In the same way that you are learning to tune into your hunger needs, keeping you physically healthy is about tuning into your body needs. By managing your stress levels and incorporating physical activity into your life in a non-obsessive, achievable and lasting way, you will be literally getting your feet back on the ground, keeping your body in good running order and reclaiming your body. Some form of physical activity – I don't mean punishing exercise regimes – can help us integrate the physical and emotional sides of ourselves.

If you've stopped dieting you may already have noticed a reduction in your stress levels and you'll be eating more healthily.

Feeling you have to conform to an ideal body shape in order to be successful, attractive and valued means pressure. Having the responsibility of shopping for and cooking food that everyone will eat and enjoy can be stressful in itself, and if, in addition, you were watching your family eat the food you cooked at the same time as depriving yourself you are likely to have been undermining your wellbeing.

The majority of women today are still carrying most of the responsibility for running a home – and holding down a job too. To put it bluntly, most women are doing too much. I was staggered to read in a women's magazine that less than 10 per cent of husbands help their working wives in the home. It's no wonder we are feeling stressed.

Stress management used to be the exclusive preserve of the male executive. Typically, their female partners and colleagues referred men to these courses – possibly because they recognized the symptoms from which they too were suffering. Women were reluctant to say they were suffering from stress. Perhaps they had struggled to climb the corporate ladder: 'admitting' to feeling under stress would leave them vulnerable in the workplace. Others recognized that taking care of their families meant they were relegating their own needs to second place. Increasingly, women are giving themselves permission to acknowledge that they too may be suffering from stress.

When we feel pressure, whether real or imagined, our bodies respond. In a short-term pressure situation our muscles tense and our breathing becomes irregular. Our brain sends the body messages to prepare for vigorous action – to fight, flee or freeze. The endocrine glands secrete hormones into the blood, and the response is automatic. We do not have to think about what to do when a car is out of control and heading our way. Without thinking, we jump out of the road fast, because the endocrine and nervous systems are activated into an alarm response.

Dieting is an on-going pressure which, like any other stress factor, causes the organs of the nervous and endocrine systems to become overstimulated with unused stress chemicals. This wears them down, and they can become diseased. It is also worth remembering that dieting is a long-term goal, and when we are under stress we can lose our ability to stick to long-term goals.

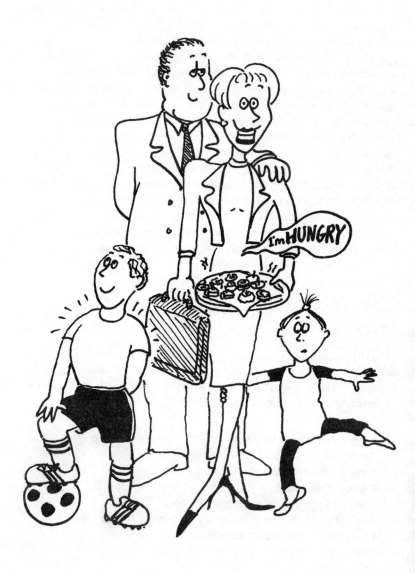

Stress interferes with our immune system, contributing to
'low-grade' illnesses such as headaches, colds, flu, constipation
and backache. We can become so accustomed to them that we

believe they are a 'normal' part of life over which we have little control.

People possess a range of coping mechanisms, some of them quite negative, to deal with the stress of dieting and body image. Dieters use avoidance to prevent themselves getting into a known stressful situation in the first place – for example, declining invitations to eat with other people for fear of losing control, or watching other people eat 'fattening' foods whilst abstaining themselves. Another avoidance technique could be not to buy clothes a size too small, to avoid the stressful feelings of failure. And, of course, the most common negative coping mechanism is trying yet another weight loss regime, video or product to avoid the stress of having to confront real feelings and issues.

Our bodies are not meant to be under constant stress. A little is good (see page 122), but too much can be lethal: living in overdrive can give us ulcers, heart attacks and other serious ailments.

Recognizing the signs and symptoms of stress

The physical symptoms listed below are generally believed to be stress-related. The starred items may well be attributable to dieting. If you can identify two or more of these physical symptoms in yourself, you may be placing yourself at risk:

- Excessive nervous energy which prevents you sitting still and relaxing
- High blood pressure
- Loss of appetite
- Wanting to eat as soon as a problem arises*
- Inability to cry, or a tendency to burst into tears easily
- Chronic diarrhoea or constipation*
- Inability to sleep*
- Constant fatigue*
- Frequent headaches*
- Needing aspirin or other medication daily
- Muscle spasm
- Feeling full even though you haven't eaten*

- Shortness of breath
- Frequent heartburn
- Proneness to fainting or nausea*
- Persistent sexual problems*
- Obesity if in conjunction with other risk factors such as high
  blood pressure

Identifying more than four of the following mental symptoms,
or a total of four mental and physical symptoms, can also indicate
that you are at risk. Again, notice how many of these symptoms
are prevalent in dieters.

- Reluctance to take a holiday or break*
- Feeling unable to talk about your problems with anyone*
- Constantly feeling uneasy*
- Feeling bored or fed up with life*
- Morbid fear of disease, especially heart disease and cancer
- Feeling rejected by your family/close friends
- Inability to have a good laugh
- Dread of the weekend approaching*
- Inability to concentrate for long*
- Inability to finish one job before starting another
- A sense of suppressed anger*
- Fear of death – yours and that of others
- Recurring feelings of being unable to cope with life
- A sense of despair for not being 'good enough'*
- Anxiousness about money
- Terror of enclosed or open spaces, heights, earthquakes,
  thunderstorms

These lists are intended to give you 'clues' to increase your stress
level awareness. If you are aware of stress in yourself you can do
something to remedy the situation or help yourself to cope.

Your progress to becoming a non-dieter may be stressful too,
but some stress in our lives is desirable so long as it doesn't become
debilitating. The challenge of aiming for new goals is stimulating,
motivating – and stressful. During the process of diet breaking
you will be developing new skills and abilities and this may make
you feel anxious, but opening your mind to new ideas is a way of

bringing variety and spice into our lives. If we don't have any stress at all we become bored, which in itself can cause stress through low stimulation. For example, many long-term unemployed and retired people suffer from low-stimulation stress.

Regrettably, some people still struggle on, ignoring all the symptoms, in the belief that conceding they are suffering from stress is synonymous with being a failure – a public announcement that they are unable to cope, not up to the job. Of course it isn't, and I hope you don't feel that. Managing your stress levels is essential to your good health. Ignoring the symptoms of stress can damage your health – and it doesn't work in the long run anyway.

And here's something else to think about: dieting can affect our natural responses to stress and anxiety. When non-dieters are put under stress they tend to eat less. This is because when we are in a stressful situation adrenalin starts to pump through our bodies to aid us in the perceived emergency, and adrenalin inhibits hunger. Studies of dieters show the opposite: dieters eat more when they are upset. The jury is still out on whether these reactions are psychological or physiological, but, either way, the effect is there.

Learning to relax

'I really need to go and relax' is our way of saying that we've had enough stress in a certain situation and want to reduce or remove the stress. It may mean sitting or lying down, reading a book, having a drink, watching televison, listening to music, going for a walk or taking some other form of exercise. For a diet breaking woman it may also mean recognizing that stress will be involved in your wanting to do something for a positive reason to achieve one of your goals, or confronting an issue that you have been avoiding for some time.

The ability to relax mentally and physically requires skills that we can learn through awareness and practice. Two skill areas that form the basis for many relaxation techniques are breathing and visualization.

Breathing exercises

When we breathe we enable oxygen to be taken up into our blood, which is then pumped around the body by the heart. When we breathe properly our bodies relax and we feel stronger.

If you look at a sleeping baby breathing you will see its tummy rising and falling as it takes in air and expels it again. I have often noticed that men seem to breathe more deeply than women, and I wonder whether this has anything to do with the fact that we women have been told for years to 'hold your tummy in'. Whatever the reason, many women do not breathe properly.

I have been practising deep breathing for the last ten or so years. Two or three times a day, whenever I think about it, I make a point of taking a few deep breaths, holding and then releasing my breath. I used to think I was a shallow breather, but then I began to realize that I breathe deeply enough but don't exhale properly. So that's what I concentrate on most. Improving my breathing has helped me feel more relaxed, and I think it has helped my circulation: I no longer get chilblains, for instance.

Here are two very simple breathing exercises. This first one has helped me to exhale. I do it any time I think about it: in the office, watching television, peeling potatoes, driving the car.

Exercise 1

- Gently blow out
- You will then automatically breathe in deeply
- Do this exercise three or four times, and then relax.

This second exercise is helpful when you need to relax. Give yourself time to do it properly – ten or fifteen minutes. Sometimes I do it at my desk, but I really prefer to lie on the floor. It's an ideal exercise to do at lunchtime. Don't do it when you are driving!

Exercise 2

- Sit or lie down and close your eyes
- Get comfortable and settle down

- Feel your body soften and relax
- Breathe out, and as you do so imagine your feelings of tension and stress leaving your body
- Breathe in – slowly – to the count of eight, and imagine feelings of calm and relaxation entering your body
- Hold your breath to the count of eight
- Breathe out to the count of eight

When you have finished this exercise, give yourself a moment or two to 'come round' rather than jumping up quickly.

If at any time during this exercise you find yourself becoming dizzy or faint, stop doing it. It may mean you are hyperventilating (over-breathing and therefore exhaling too much carbon dioxide, which causes dizziness and fainting). One way to deal with it is to breathe into a paper bag a few times, which should stop any dizziness. But if this is a persistent problem for you, it would be wise to speak to your GP.

Creative visualization

These days many people use the technique of creative visualization. Sports teams and management consultants, for instance, use it to enhance performance, while health professionals use it to help empower patients suffering from illnesses such as cancer and AIDS. Sales and marketing trainers tell their students to 'visualize' success, to see themselves clinching the deal, shaking hands, signing the contract and so on.

I use it in some of my training courses, and I use it for myself too. For example, when I am going to take part in a television interview I will visualize myself being relaxed, smiling, answering the questions and furthering the debate – rather than freezing up or losing my cool. I find this helps me to relax and stops me frightening myself with all the cameras, lights and other media paraphernalia. I know I am more likely to get the results I want when I approach tricky situations in a positive frame of mind.

Creative visualization is similar to daydreaming. When we visualize we make a deliberate decision to use our daydreaming ability, but are much more focussed about its content and objective.

You can use creative visualization for any situation that you find stressful. If you are going out to dinner tonight, picture yourself looking relaxed, moving confidently, smiling and enjoying the food in a guilt-free way. See yourself eating in the diet breaking way:

- Being in tune with your body and hunger
- Selecting the food you fancy
- Tasting and enjoying the food
- Eating until you are full
- Assertively declining food when you've had enough

Recognize the positive thoughts and feelings that go with this visualization, and hang on to them to carry with you into the real situation. Have another run-through just before your evening starts. Creative visualizations can be enjoyable in their own right!

This technique is one that improves with practice, and at the beginning your picture may be dim. However, just like turning up the brightness control on the television, we can turn up the brightness control on our visualizations to make them clearer and sharper.

If you have never done creative visualization before, you may feel foolish or consider it a waste of time. On the first few occasions I too felt uncomfortable and embarrassed. But my friend Bea Pike, who is an osteopath and works with me on stress management courses, talked me through the visualization a couple of times and then I was able to do it by myself. I relaxed and closed my eyes, and she told me a story or described a scenario which I then visualized. So if you find it hard to get to grips with visualization, why not ask a friend to help you?

Massage

Another useful relaxation technique, massage stimulates the flow of blood, assists in clearing away waste products from muscle cells and reduces muscular tension and associated pain.

It can also be valuable on an emotional level. The physical contact between two people can in itself be comforting, while massage can help reduce emotional tensions and anxiety and replace them with a sense of calm and trust. The person giving the massage can also benefit from the sense of touch and the pleasure of helping someone in a direct and personal way. If you have a poor body image, massage will help you to get used to having your body touched (or to touching it yourself).

You can, of course, massage any part of the body, but for stress the most effective parts are the neck, shoulders and forehead.

- Try to avoid interruptions (e.g. turn the phone off and close the door)
- Make sure you and your partner are comfortable and warm
- Massage should never be painful
- Try to keep the rhythm of strokes smooth, and always work towards the heart
- Always repeat strokes on both sides of the body
- Avoid any varicose veins
- Concentrate on what you are doing
- Give yourself time – don't rush
- Keep your breathing steady
- If you find it hard to be touched you may find it easier to start with massaging your hands, feet and head

Get to know yourself better

Close your eyes and visualize any stressful situation in order to relive and even feel the emotional and physical sensations that accompanied it. In the lead-up to these situations you will start to feel anxious anticipation of the event by way of low-intensity cues such as tummy wobbles or sweaty palms. As you tune in to these sensations you will be in a better position to stop and ask yourself, 'Do I really want to put myself under this kind of pressure?' before it becomes too difficult to extricate yourself.

Perhaps facets of your dieting behaviour cause you stress. If you think about it, every individual is 'responsible' for his or her own stress. Being invited out by friends to a restaurant will be a pleasure to your partner but may give you immense anxiety. If you have a love/hate relationship with food, if you dread having to eat a full meal in front of others because of your fear of losing control, you will experience a range of emotions and physical symptoms that are stressful. At the time you may not even realize it is happening, perhaps through denial or the successful ways you have found to cope with the situation.

The problem-solving approach

You will already have been weighing up the pros and cons of dieting behaviour, and if you have started to adopt some of the ideas in this book you are undoubtedly reducing the number of stressful situations in your life. If you are eating regularly and responding to your physical hunger needs, for example, it is likely that you are experiencing fewer mood swings and no longer feeling you're living on the edge – only one bite away from failure.

So let's look at handling the stressful situations that arise from diet breaking. However well you are doing in developing a positive image, if you have not been swimming in a public pool for years (because you don't feel your body is attractive enough) it is reasonable to expect the situation to feel threatening at first. Visualize yourself going to the pool, and tune into the physical and emotional symptoms that arise. Don't deny their presence. Where do they come from? Can you remember a similar situation in the past when you experienced these same feelings? So, what happened?

It's possible you felt embarrassment because of a rude remark or a feeling that people were staring at you, and now, twenty years later, you feel embarrassed again at the thought of a similar situation. You have learned to react in this way, but now it's time to start unlearning that behaviour.

- How important is going swimming to you?
- Think of what you will do to solve the problem – not how you will be
- List the problems you will encounter *en route* to achieving this
- Produce a range of strategies to increase your confidence, such as treating yourself to a nice new swimming costume
- Produce a range of strategies to reduce the perceived impact of the 'outside world' (e.g. strangers looking at you). Go with a friend, or as part of a group

- Take strength from others who have managed to overcome their embarrassment. If possible, find out how they did it. If not, watch them in action and copy their behaviour
- Look at your strategies and prioritize them from most to least practical
- Try out the most practical and achievable strategy
- Break your strategy down into steps
- Take one step at a time

Expressing our feelings

Being able to express our feelings appropriately is a great stress reliever. If we're feeling sad and unhappy, being able to cry usually helps us feel better. There are healing properties in tears, and they release the tension. I know of some women who feel unable to cry when they feel sad but watch weepy videos and get their release that way. Listening to sad music can help. So can talking to people.

As women, many of us have been socialized into being 'nice', which means hiding (or swallowing) our 'nasty' feelings. Remind yourself that your feelings are natural and legitimate. Getting out of the diet mentality can leave a residue of sadness or anger – about the energy, time and money wasted.

Try not to keep your feelings bottled up inside you: find ways to deal with it. Suppressing your anger is not good for you, and it usually breaks out when you least want it to – aimed sometimes at the wrong people, and sometimes towards ourselves. There are times when we all feel like exploding because we feel so angry. Good health management is not about denying your anger, it's about finding ways to express and honour it in a way that helps you.

Talking the issue through with the other person or people involved is a good idea. It helps reinforce your personal power, and if it is done in an honest and non-blaming way it enables both parties to gain insight from the situation. In addition, talking to people who are not involved can help you shed light on the situation, perhaps seeing things from a different point of view.

On occasions when you feel like exploding, just express it – get that anger out of your body. Try screaming in the broom cupboard, bashing the rugs with a carpet beater, jumping up and down or stamping your feet. One method I especially like the sound of is the one told me by a woman who buys second-hand china in jumble sales and markets: when she feels angry she gets a pile and systematically smashes them.

This exercise is great when you feel you want to shout at someone, or when circumstances and events are mounting up unbearably. I invite participants in my workshops to try it, and I use it myself when I feel angry with a person or situation and I am not able to deal with it smoothly – such as nameless officials when I have a query with something like a gas or telephone bill. Your feelings may be legitimate and shouting at people may be rewarding, but it is not always recommended! This exercise bridges the gap:

- Find a room or space where you can be yourself and remain undisturbed
- Cross your arms loosely in front of your chest (as if you're about to embark on that old chestnut: I must, I must, improve my bust)
- Picture in your mind's eye the person, product or advertisement which you reacted against so angrily, or the man who leered at you in the street
- Breathe in deeply
- Using your full voice, as you swing your elbows back, shout: 'GET OFF MY BACK!'
- Repeat this over and over until you feel energized or exhausted – either way I always feel better, because I've got the rotten feelings out of my shoulders.

Finding other things to do

I am not advocating avoidance of a difficult situation, but having an interest or project that requires your time and attention and gives you pleasure helps you put the problem in perspective and therefore reduce stress. The crux of the diet mentality is that it keeps you inward-looking, so any activity that helps take you 'out of yourself' or that helps you focus on your skills and abilities can reduce the stresses around bodyism and the tyranny of thinness.

Physical activity

'Women of all sizes not only have a right to play and be physically active without focusing on weight loss as a goal, but also have a right to see positive images of themselves in action,' say Pat Lyons and Debby Burgard in *Great Shape*. The present obsession with fitness is not about health but about striving for the perfect body. For men that means slim and muscular, with pert bottoms; for women it means thin – the thinner the better.

Dieting, thinness, health and fitness are all interwoven in the big guilt trip. Any woman watching daytime television is encouraged to become a health and diet zombie. We are required to prance around our living rooms at breakfast time doing stretching exercises, and mid-morning we can diet and exercise with another guru. We can attend step aerobics classes or sponsored fat-burning sessions in the lunch hour. With the right mix of physical jerks and a good measure of willpower we can spot-reduce those nasty areas of fat on our tummies, thighs and bottoms.

If you feel alienated by all this, take heart – you're not alone. And if you find yourself trapped in an obsessive exercise regime in order to slim, take care, because you may be doing yourself more harm than good.

Responding to yet another external cue doesn't work. Incorporating more physical activity into our lives is not sustainable if we have not made it a permanent lifestyle change. Physical activity done regularly and at a comfortable level is an excellent method of managing our stress levels and improving our physical and mental health. But let's put fitness into perspective: it is only one aspect of the healthy person, not the be-all and end-all. You don't live any longer if you are a superfit sportsperson.

Studies have shown that if you're fit you'll live longer. Linda Omichinski, an accredited fitness leader, says exercise doesn't have to be punishingly strenuous but only at a level where your pulse rate is raised so as to exercise your heart and lungs. In fact, the higher the intensity you work at, especially if it's irregular, the more likely you are to sustain serious injury or, worse still, suffer a heart attack. The equivalent of a brisk thirty-minute walk a day is enough to increase your odds of living a long and healthy life. She points out that ordinary active living – such as walking up stairs, gardening, parking your car a little further away and walking to your destination – can use up 25 per cent of your calorie intake.

No pain, no gain? No way!

So forget all the hype about burning off fat through exercise, and 'no pain, no gain'; it's misleading. If you lose weight fast it's just water, and during exercise we need to be constantly replenishing the water in our bodies to prevent dehydration. You don't burn off fat but use up your carbohydrate stores, certainly during the first thirty minutes of exercise. If you're dieting as well, after that point you will be depleting lean muscle tissue, which will leave you weakened and will be difficult to replace later.

Punishing exercise regimes hook into old feelings of not being good enough – and therefore we've got to be whipped into shape. When it's hurting like crazy, how can it be enjoyable? If it isn't enjoyable, how can we stick to it? We won't – and we don't!

Exercise isn't in fact a very effective way of losing fat although it may prevent you from gaining it. In *You Don't have to Diet* Tom Sanders and Peter Bazalgette say that to lose 1 kg of fat (2.2 pounds) you would need to do something like cycling for sixteen hours! Low-intensity activities like walking, swimming or cycling (jogging exerts three times your body weight on your joints and muscles), or any other activity in your life which raises your pulse above normal and is done regularly, provides these benefits:

- Better appetite control
- Hunger signals between your stomach and your brain work better
- Less constipation/better digestion
- A more naturally active intestine
- Reduction of stress and tension
- Secretion of chemical endorphins which act as a relaxant
- Decreased effects of stress hormones
- More energy
- Stimulates your heart and lungs to increase oxygen and nutrient delivery around your body
- Stimulates feelings of exhilaration through enjoyment and secretion of endorphins, the body's natural painkillers

- Increased metabolic rate for up to six hours afterwards
- Increased feelings of self-worth, confidence, self-acceptance and achievement
- Improves joint problems and reduces muscle cramps
- Lowers blood pressure
- Makes blood vessels more elastic
- Reduces deposition of fat in arteries
- Lowers blood sugar levels
- Makes you sleep better

By exercising consistently, at a comfortable level, you will develop an increased capacity to work with less effort. You'll be using less from your carbohydrate store, and more fat, for energy.

Suitable pursuits for ladies

Exercise for women is a relatively new idea. Less than a hundred years ago genteel ladies were being reared to be little more than delicate, passively frail wives – amusing little pastimes for their husbands after a hard day's work out in the real world. It was not considered ladylike to do terribly much – and certainly not physical exercise, where one might break out into a sweat (sorry, perspiration!).

Of course, to maintain these high standards it helped to have a bevy of working-class women around to cook and clean, milk cows, pick potatoes, scrub floors, make fires and carry coal, which meant they were getting all the exercise they needed. And because the working-class women were so coarse anyway, it didn't matter that they sweated!

Not surprisingly, all this inactivity and boredom impaired the health of many upper middle-class women. So doctors began recommending 'suitable' recreational activities that enabled the ladies to be outside enjoying the fresh air and socializing with others from the same class. Croquet, tennis, archery and swimming were considered acceptable for a lady – provided she wore appropriate clothing and stopped these activities during the 'difficult time of the month'.

Around the turn of the century bicycles became the craze. There were concerns about the appropriateness of cycling and the damage that could be done to women (by the saddles), but women ignored this prejudiced rubbish and started cycling for pleasure and as a form of transport.

Things have improved a lot since then, of course, although professional sportswomen have had to fight hard to gain the same respect as their male counterparts and equal prize money. But sports and physical activities for women and girls are still not as much a part of daily life as they are for men and boys. With the exception of special events such as the annual hockey international at Wembley tennis at Wimbledon and major athletics meetings, we don't get coverage of women's sport on radio and television. We are still a long way from switching on to watch an all-female *Match of the Day*. Consequently, exercise is not part of the collective female psyche – it is not considered a normal, everyday activity.

Let's change all that – but in our own way

At school, when we played games people would have to pick teams. I was always one of the last to be picked. It was OK when a friend of mine was choosing, or better still when I had the power and was the selector, but otherwise it was a nightmare for me. Nobody wanted me in their team.

Once, when I was about eight years old, my family went to a wedding. I remember feeling embarrassed seeing my mother dancing. I had never seen her dance before. In fact I had never seen my mother do any form of exercise other than working – either in our home or in someone else's. It wasn't until years later that I recalled this memory, wondering whether it was in some way related to my telling myself I couldn't dance 'because I was uncoordinated and had no sense of rhythm'.

I am not a natural wallflower and did not enjoy being one, sitting round the edge of the room looking at others enjoying themselves. I could dance, and yet I feared being laughed at. I had not learnt to move and to enjoy my body, but I was too concerned about what other people might be thinking of me. When I danced I felt self-conscious. If I enjoyed it I felt embarrassed. It has been hard to get out of this terrible trap. Walking, gardening, going to the gym and swimming regularly have all helped me. The more I move my body, the more I am able to feel it and respond to its needs. And I like it more, too.

Many women tell me they feel foolish about taking up any form of exercise, believing they won't be any good. I suggest they start doing it simply because they want to, for the enjoyment of the activity – not to be good at it. Nobody can be good at something first off.

One of the first activities I took up was swimming. I started going first thing in the morning. Often I didn't feel like it because I was still half asleep and grumpy. Yet, ten or a dozen gentle lengths later, I would get out of the pool feeling better: chirpy, chatty and alive. Then I started going after work – which was a real drag. I didn't feel like it because I was tired and ready to put my feet up. Yet when I pushed myself that little bit, I would feel great afterwards – ready for the next round of the day.

Apart from helping us to feel better, exercise helps us to look more attractive. It gives us more vitality and tones our muscles – whatever our size. There is nothing more attractive than a woman with energy and zest for life.

My body generally feels healthier and more efficient now that I am keeping it in better working order. It has also helped my aching back through strengthening my leg and stomach muscles. After my slow, tentative start with swimming I went on to a gym, which I now attend two or three times a week.

I feel a great sense of achievement after a particularly negative experience at a previous health club. I went swimming there, but needed three months to build up enough courage to go into the gym. I was fighting my own lack of confidence and a club culture that oozed competition, slenderness and 'glamour'. I didn't feel I would ever feel comfortable being with bone-thin women dressed in skin-tight lycra one-pieces, who were furiously over-exercising and who applied their make-up before they went into the gym. So I recommend you to look around first, and find a place where you feel comfortable and that is going to work for you. Don't be persuaded into thinking that a trendy place is the best place to be.

Before taking up exercise, some people go out and buy expensive gear to help them get started. That can be a bit like people declaring they are going to stop smoking when they've finished their last duty-frees, or like women who feel better for making the decision to diet. In other words they are declarations for the future – emollients for the guilt. You don't need to spend a fortune on the latest super-duper workout kit. You don't need sexy lycra all-in-one jogging suits, gossamer swimwear or very expensive equipment. Be more modest. Wear comfortable clothes.

Don't take up exercise to try to stop yourself feeling guilty. Guilt is not helpful for anything, because it is not a motivator. It serves only as a persecutor. And don't buy lots of equipment. You may be wasting your money. More than half of all training equipment bought for the home isn't used within six months of purchase.

If getting started is the hardest thing, staying motivated is the next hardest. So it is very important that whatever you do it is for you – the benefits are for you, and so are the pleasure and the pay-offs.

Are you thinking, 'I'd like to do some exercise but I don't have enough time to do all the things I do already?' If so, it might be a good idea to think about what you are spending your time on. Time is a resource; don't waste it doing only things you don't want to do. Spend a few minutes thinking about the following:

- How many hours do you spend working each day: (a) at home? (b) at work?
- How much time do you have for yourself or for leisure each day?
- Of your daily leisure time, how much is spent: (a) watching TV (b) on a social activity, e.g. talking to friends/family (c) relaxing, e.g. bath, reading, knitting (d) on physical activity?
- Do you really, honestly, want to do more physical activity?
- If you answered 'No', consider your three main reasons why not.
- Are they reasons that you might overcome? If so, how might you overcome them?
- Or are you just not attracted to physical activity? If this is the case, it is better to accept the fact rather than flog yourself with 'ought to's', which never work for long anyway. 'Want to's' are always more successful.
- If you answered 'Yes', what would be the pay-offs for you doing more physical activity?
- Of the above leisure pursuits, which could you spend less time on?

- Which physical activity do you fancy that could fit into this 'saved' time?
- Is it realistic? If not, find something else that is.
- What do you need to do to get yourself started?
- What do you need to do to keep yourself motivated?
- How might you stop yourself from continuing the activity?
- Who could help/support you do more physical activity?
- Who might try to hinder your plans?
- Think of ways to circumvent/negotiate their hindrances.
  (Adapted from Melpomene Institute Questionnaire).

Looking at your answers

After spending a bit of time on these questions you should be clearer about whether you really want to become more physically active, and if so what you want to try. You will also be clearer about your personal blockages – how you might demotivate yourself, how others might try to get in the way of your plans too – and how to prevent them.

You will also have squashed that old excuse 'lack of time'. I believe we find time to do the things we want to do. It is better to say, 'I choose not to do more physical activity, because I don't want to' than to carry on inventing excuses. You don't need excuses. It is easier to start accepting and liking ourselves when we get to know ourselves.

Try the activity first and see if you like it. If table tennis is not for you, move on and try something else. Keep experimenting until you find something that suits you. If you decide to join a class or group activity, make sure you find one that is at the right level for you. Nothing will demotivate you more quickly than being unable to keep up with the rest of the participants. The idea is to find activities that will work for you and that you will enjoy doing – for yourself.

When you have found what suits you, then – and only then – is it time to buy the jogging shoes, tennis skirt, caving suit and helmet, whatever. Like clothes that are too tight, a wet suit will not encourage you to go deep sea diving if you don't like the water. This way you may be saving yourself a fortune on discarded outfits, and you can buy to suit your needs when you are clearer about the particular activity you want to do.

Watching a group of middle-aged Americans shopping in Kensington High Street got me thinking about whether the current fashion to wear tracksuits and trainers out in the street is about helping us to feel we are being active. The outfits create an illusion of activity.

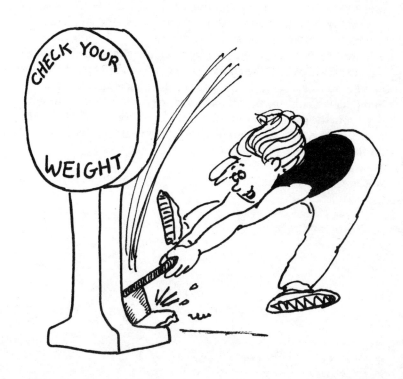

Any activity should be undertaken for you – because you enjoy it and because it makes you feel good. Experts suggest we do a combination of aerobic and anaerobic exercise. Anaerobics are exercises that don't use up lots of oxygen, such as stretching, mobility and flexibility, as well as those for muscle strengthening. They are recommended to improve overall fitness. Aerobic exercising means an activity such as running or cycling, which increases your heartbeat and makes you breathe fast and harder. If you run regularly your heart, lungs and circulation will expand

and strengthen, your blood and oxygen supply will improve, and so in turn will other functions in your body.

But do remember that if you have any medical complications or believe yourself to be unwell in any way you ought to check with your doctor before you take up physical exercise. You may need to search for a health professional who is not in the diet mentality themselves and has up-to-date knowledge of the health risks of physical activity for those with a perceived 'weight problem'.

Finally, another quick and easy way to increase your physical activity is to incorporate more movement into your daily life. Make a point of walking up the stairs to work rather than taking the lift, and go out for a walk every day. Have a dance around at home. Stand up to do the ironing. Stand up to answer the phone. Do some digging in the garden, or mow the lawn. Don't wait until your friend comes to do it with you, or until you've had your hair done, or until all the housework is done, or until. . . . Start today!

7

Putting Your Best Foot Forward

A journalist who was writing an article about dieting asked me if I believed Dawn French when she said she really liked her body. I don't know Dawn French, so I have no idea of knowing, but if you watch the way she moves she certainly gives the impression of being at home in her body. Perhaps the journalist's disbelief had more to do with her feelings towards her own body than it had to do with Dawn French.

When we suffer from negative body image we develop highly tuned antennae – every picture jumps up and hits us in the eye, every conversation rings in our ears, twisting and turning, telling us we're ugly, fat, hopeless. You become a prisoner in your own personal hell-cell. I know, because I've been there, and it is a terrible place to be. So in this chapter we shall be covering:

- projecting ourselves positively
- making the most of our appearance

Improving our body image

Diet Breakers supporter Cathy Shaw sent this poem to me.

Here is a diet
– I think you should try it –
It differs a bit from the norm
Just ration your intake
Of images which make
You yearn for a more petite form

This is a diet
– I think you should try it –

Cut down on the hate and self-loathing
Reduce your consumption
Of media assumptions
That what counts is the size of your clothing

This is a diet
– All women should try it –
Deny yourself nothing – it's radical!
Just try and resist
Your belief in the myth
That you must be an eight stone fanatical!

It is rare to find a woman who has a positive body image and feels good about her body. Those few whom I have come across have usually done a lot of work on themselves to undo all the negative messages and distorted images we have absorbed throughout our lives.

Finding the source of our dislike

Perhaps your sister was considered more physically attractive than you. Perhaps you were always seen as the short one in your family. Maybe a well-meaning but misguided mother poked fun at your thighs. A number of women will have been sexually abused as children. When you consider the multitude of reasons that result in us hating and being ashamed of our bodies, how facile it is to imagine that a diet product could be the answer to our problems. It just adds to our torment and torture.

Responses to DB questionnaires show that women have definite body areas which they dislike/hate, and which seem to change depending on our age.

Typically in our dieting careers we will have been attracted to 'fib and lie' diet books that tell us how to spot reduce our 'nasty' areas. Along with our faces, these are the body parts that women have cosmetic surgery to 'correct'.

Our emotions are carried in our bodies, and when we feel ashamed of our bodies we express our shame in the way we move and behave. We 'hide' various parts of ourselves through our body language and our clothes; we cover our belly by folding our arms across it, we cover our face with our hands or our hair, we sit and stand hunched up so as not to take up too much space, and we wear clothes designed to obliterate rather than celebrate.

We might develop a 'hang-dog' posture with drooping head and shoulders and shuffle along in a manner which apologizes for our very existence. Poor body posture affects our breathing, depriving our body of oxygen which is essential for health, energy, vitality and confidence. And the less confident we feel, the more shallowly we breathe. Walking around like this for a period of time can result in aches and pains, which too many of us accept as normal rather than as a sign that something isn't right.

Judy wrote to Diet Breakers:

My self-esteem increases dependent on who I am with/what I am doing. At the moment I am in a steady relationship which sometimes serves to increase my self-esteem about my body and self, but only when I am pleased with it myself. If I am unhappy with myself/body my partner does not affect the way I perceive myself despite lots of positive statements from him about my figure.

It is essential to investigate the source of this self-inflicted hurt in order to understand how it came about and to begin learning to love and appreciate ourselves. Another woman wrote:

I think my success is due to the fact that it was something I want for myself and my health. I was always on diets because other people wanted me to lose weight. At the back of it all I was led to believe my sole (soul) purpose was to be attractive to men, which hindered me by making me angry. People could not see there was a lot more to me than my figure. I am in fact a sensitive, artistic, intelligent person.

Reject comparison – choose celebration

When asked to draw outlines of themselves, most women think they are larger than they really are. Being larger is almost always felt to be negative. A number of women have told me they *must* do something because they are bigger than their husbands. I ask them whether they would expect their husbands to take steroids and go to the gym to get bigger. To date every woman has replied 'no' – they would not expect their husbands to go to such lengths to change their size and shape. So we women inflict harsher standards on ourselves than we do on others. The paradox is that when we feel bad about ourselves and/or our bodies we may turn to food to comfort, punish or anaesthetize ourselves.

When you are in the company of other women, do you compare yourself to them? Do you find yourself scanning the room, sizing and grading the women, trying to find where you are in the pecking order? It is a gruelling activity which doesn't really achieve much. By constantly comparing yourself to other women you are distancing yourself from them, which further adds to feelings of isolation and insecurity. And if you do, what does it really tell you? We don't compare a Palomino horse with a Shetland pony, or a blue tit with a parrot. So why do we compare ourselves with other women?

How can we measure the beauty of Michele Pfeiffer against the beauty of Alice Walker or Emma Thompson? Or Bea Arthur against Maya Angelou or the Duchess of Kent? And what is beauty anyway? There is more to beauty than meets the eye – it really isn't just about how we look. As the saying goes, you can't judge a sausage by its skin. Nor should you be fooled into believing that all other women have everything sussed. The way you see her could be very different from the way she sees herself. As Betty wrote to Diet Breakers: 'A low weight does not always equal a high life'!

OK, so you might initially feel better if you come across a woman whom you consider less attractive than you. But the chances of this become increasingly rare, because the more you make these comparisons the harsher judge do you become, giving yourself more self-doubts and needless envy. Remember:

- There is no shortage of beauty.
- Other women's beauty does not make you less beautiful.

What's the point of thinking, 'I want to look like her' or even 'I don't want to look like her'? You don't look like her. You look like you. You are not meant to look like Jasmin LeBon, Oprah Winfrey, Sharon Stone or anybody else. You are you, and that's good enough. So let's move away from the constant competition with other women. Make a point of looking for and celebrating the beauty in yourself and others. We all have it.

There's a Venus in us all

Liz wrote to Diet Breakers about how she changed her feelings about her own and other women's bodies:

I'm neither fat nor thin any more, but I've been both and I know how it feels. Fat isn't just a description, its a moral condemnation, an insult to character as well as appearance. It stands for everything we despise and fear to be. I've suffered because of this, physically and emotionally, and so have thousands of other intelligent, attractive and healthy women.

Our society is wrong about fat: its ideas must be challenged and overthrown. Seeing the beauty of non-thin women takes a little time, because of the instant condemnation we have all been taught at the sight of a body with any flesh on it.

You have to adjust your eyes and fight against everything you've believed. A few years ago somebody bought me a poster of Botticelli's *Birth of Venus*, which shows the goddess of love coming in from the sea in great magesty on a huge conch shell surrounded by worshipping attendants. I'd never looked at it closely before, but I hung her by my bed and found myself gazing at her each night before I went to sleep.

She is naked, and her hair winds around her and drifts in the wind. The movement of sea and air about her heightens the voluptuous smoothness, grace and movement of her body, and you long to reach out and touch her skin. Everything about the painting is soft – the pink shell, the hazy blue-green of the sea, the edges of the clouds, the billowing robes of her attendants, and, most interesting of all, Venus herself.

After all, this is the goddess of love, Botticelli's vision of the most seductive and alluring of women, but she is startlingly different from the flat-stomached, narrow-hipped images of sexuality we recognize from catwalks and advertising hoardings. She radiates a sexual vitality we have sadly learned to associate only with thin bodies, and one look at her shows us clearly what we have lost.

I thought she was beautiful – and then I realized that she looks like me! It took a while to see past all the things we're told every day about beauty and thinness and sexuality, but Venus changed my attitude.

I'd spent years feeling grateful to the men in my life for not minding my imperfections, when I was not imperfect at all. Thinking about it, if I look like Venus, that makes them pretty damn lucky!

Only the ones who realize this stand a chance, these days, and I've never had so many offers. It just goes to show what confidence does, and that was something my diets never gave me. Botticelli could teach us all a thing or two, and it's about time we learned, so that beautiful women don't waste their lives believing they're ugly and defective, and we can be free to celebrate the Venus in us all.

Elaine, another Diet Breakers correspondent, also found positive pictures useful:

I made a point of collecting postcards from all the major museums of images of women, especially ideals of desirability. I was really turned on to see my body pretty much exactly the way a sexual woman has been imagined by men throughout most of Western history: soft, rounded, blowsy, opulent. I was fat, but I was shapely and strong, because I always maintained my exercise and activity.

We need to get away from the idea of valuing women purely on a looks basis, because it makes us insecure and devalues our qualities and abilities. When you are with other women, don't look at them to find faults. Look for their positive qualities – in their characters as well as physically. When you notice something favourable or are impressed, tell her. Be specific – tell her you like her sense of style or the way she wears her hair or the way she handled a particular situation. The more you look for beauty, goodness, skills, whatever, the more you notice them and, unsurprisingly, the more you can learn. Watch how the women you admire and respect behave.

It's show time!

Do you check your reflection in every shop window to see if you are OK? Are you concerned when you pass a man and don't get that look in the eye or nod of approval? I call it the monkey walk. I don't remember anyone ever telling me about it or getting any lessons in how to do it, yet I did it for years.

We walk down the street and as we pass a man we look at him to see how he looks at us. If he looks appreciatively we feel good, and if he doesn't, or if he ignores us, it's a needle prick into our self-esteem. It is as though every encounter with every man in every street is a little test of us being OK.

Now, most of these men mean absolutely nothing to us. Their only relevance to us is that they are passing a particular spot on this planet at the same time as us. And yet we hold ourselves up for scrutiny, comment and approval to this stranger.

It you recognize yourself here, take heart! No matter how long you've been doing this, there is a brilliantly easy solution. This is not a natural behaviour, it is a learned behaviour. All you have to do is learn a different behaviour, and this is what you do.

As you walk past a man, don't look at him. Just go about your business as though he wasn't there. This way you neatly side-step any argy-bargy about feeling attractive enough. It might seem a little odd or a bit unfriendly at first. It isn't, it's assertive. The more you do it, the easier it becomes. You can choose who you want to be friendly with. You don't need approval from others to feel all right. Try it. It really works.

Down with denigration!

Some of the messages from our personal megaphone have been whirling around our heads, fermenting, for years. Others are regularly updated for us by other people. Sometimes, even more confusingly, we find ourselves in a terrible double bind, trying to run with the fox as we hunt with the hounds, perpetuating the message – and apparently benefiting from it – and at the same time we are victims. During a breakfast meeting at the Savoy, I watched a senior executive play with her all-fruit breakfast and describe her body as slug-like. She works for one of the largest publishers of diet books!

Denigrating terms such as flab, balloon and beached whale are common parlance and remain largely unchallenged. Those with vested interests in promoting their product – the media who have bought into the tyranny of thinness, and individuals themselves with personal, unresolved issues about their own body image – churn this stuff out with annoying regularity.

When you read about a female celebrity whose weight has 'ballooned', what picture do you get? A body whose weight goes up and down faster than an elevator in the Empire State Building? A balloon is made of gossamer-thin, pliable rubber. You only have to breathe into it for it to get bigger and bigger – and, by implication, you only have to eat to get bigger and bigger. When we hear a woman described as a 'beached whale' we are encouraged to see a pathetically dehydrated creature stranded on a beach, unable to move. How dare they liken women to beached whales and balloons in such a hurtful way! It is hard to have a thought without words. Visually descriptive words create powerful images which stick.

- If you catch yourself either thinking or using denigrating or unkind words, don't be hard on yourself. Be pleased that you noticed yourself doing it and resolve to take the word or words out of your vocabulary.
- If your friends use such terms, talk to them about why it is important for us to eliminate them from our language. Tell them about the harm these words do. But don't forget that, unless they are sympathetic to your aim of diet breaking, they may not understand first time around.
- Refuse to play the game of: 'You look really good, you've lost weight', so as not to perpetuate the diet mentality and size prejudice.

Feeling is important

Contrary to the hype and lies, a thinner body does not guarantee a positive body image. How we feel about our bodies is more important than how we actually look. To enjoy a positive body image, we need to *feel* lovely.

Deborah is 5 foot 6 inches tall and weighs 9 stone 10 pounds (136 pounds). She dieted for fourteen years and said, 'I have had difficulty accepting myself as I am. I felt that if I was thinner, then I would feel more attractive within myself.' In 1991 she dieted down to 7 stone 11 pounds (109 pounds) yet 'still felt unattractive and fat.'

Dieting is not the answer to feeling lovely. It might initially help you to feel better, because at least you are doing something about the horrible feelings, but feeling lovely does not result from depriving and punishing yourself. To feel lovely we have to get our bodies and minds working for us rather than against us, which means starting from where we are now.

- Criticism and disgust with yourself are not helpful – or true. You are not disgusting. Nobody is disgusting.
- Self-loathing is not at all helpful because it holds us back from finding ways to heal our wounds, change our attitudes and improve our self-image.
- Self-hatred is not natural. It is learned. You can learn to accept and love yourself.

Poor body image can and does prevent us from doing what we want to do, and we can use it as an excuse to hold us back. Growing and developing means travelling in uncharted waters which can be frightening, so we stay safe by blaming our bodies and ducking the challenge. Or perhaps we fear being our true self.

- Take a moment to close your eyes and imagine how you would be if you were your true, powerful, lovely self.
- Do you see yourself as confident and assertive, or are you abusing your power?
- Think back to where these images may have come from.
- Now think of a woman who is confident and assertive who is not abusing her power. Which qualities and characteristics do you both share?

The power of imagination

Our body image is a product of our imagination. It therefore stands to reason that if we use our imaginations differently our body image will be different. Making the effort to create positive images of yourself – real or imagined – can really help. My husband is a keen potholer and carries photographs of his expeditions around with him. In one he is dangling on a rope 300 feet below ground, and in the other he is squeezing out of a cave entrance with a big grin of accomplishment on his face. He says he gets pleasure, comfort and strength from glancing at the photographs when he is feeling low or having self-doubts. Through looking at the photographs he manages to get in touch with past feelings of pride and inner strength, and he transfers those feelings to the tricky situation he is presently facing.

If you have a photograph of yourself that you like, you could carry it with you. Make sure it is one that looks like you now – not twenty years ago or when you were a different shape or weight. If you don't have a photograph that you like, think back to an occasion where you feel you looked great – perhaps you were going to a party or for an interview. Memorize that image of yourself and bring it to the front of your mind when you need it.

Jane, a woman who had been sexually abused as a child of four, wrote to me about her eating disorder and her relationship with her body. 'Needless to say, I hated my body, hated people looking at me, hated my first husband touching me, hated myself.' But things changed for the better, she continued:

By a stroke of luck I came into contact with a psychologist who ran a survivor group for adult victims of child sex abuse. I began to realize that the answer was to overcome the effects the abuse had on me. I had to deal with the root of the problem rather than what was on the surface.

Last year I divorced my husband and for the first time lived alone. It was just a little bedsit with a skylight – nobody could look in. I had by then come to terms with food and no longer binged, but I no longer wanted to deny myself anything either. I ate when I was hungry or simply fancied the taste of anything, and ate anything I wanted.

My body image still bothered me. Living alone now, I decided to tackle it. It was summer and warm. From the moment I got home, I undressed and then walked around the flat naked. It felt uncomfortable at first to look at the folds of fat and skin, but I slowly began to accept it and then to like myself. I watched TV naked, cooked naked, washed the dishes naked and didn't get dressed until the next morning. I have a partner now who adores my body, and I am at peace with myself. I have thrown away my diet books, refuse to buy women's magazines which are so heavily spiced with 'Twenty Ways to Flatten Your Tum' or 'How to Be Seductive to Get Your Man', and now revel in my own glorious individuality.

Body image: mirror exercises

When we hide parts of our bodies we can forget what they look like, or focus only on negative elements. We see ourselves as objects – we stand back and look at our image reflected in the mirror.

The purpose of these next two exercises is to help you familiarize yourself with you, and to start seeing yourself rather than looking and judging. I have known some women become tearful when they allow themselves to see and get to know themselves better. Do your utmost to suspend judgement, and just allow yourself to see.

Good morning, good morning . . .

- Using a hand mirror or the bathroom mirror, make a point of looking into your eyes and seeing yourself in the mornings. Nod or smile in acknowledgement if you feel like it.

The more I see you

To help us start appreciating and feeling relaxed in our bodies again, we need to get reacquainted with them. You can do this using a full-length mirror. A gradual increase in familiarity over time is going to work best. Remember also that if you do feel negative about different parts of yourself you will probably be adopting a posture which emphasizes this.

- Breathe deeply and evenly.
- Loosen up and get some movement and flexibility in your body by stretching gently and shaking your arms and legs.
- Stand tall. Feel your physical 'presence' positively.
- When you are ready, take a look at yourself in the mirror.

In the same way that you would increase distance over a period of time when training as a runner, increase your exposure time as you train to appreciate and accept your body.

Diets are unsexy

Living with a poor body image can be tantamount to living in solitary confinement. Many women tell me they are desperate to be close to and intimate with other people, yet feel unable to relax and allow themselves to be. A poor body image can wreck people's sex lives: feeling ashamed of our bodies inhibits us. So we hold ourselves back, deny our needs, suppress our desires, pull our tummies in as we try to have an orgasm, or undress in the dark, fearful of being seen in an unflattering light without our clothes and our make-up.

Intimacy is about sharing our bodies and our vulnerability. It isn't possible to have good, enjoyable sex and still look like you stepped out of a fashion magazine or a television studio. If you have been waiting to get thinner before taking a lover, bear in mind Deborah's experience at 7 stone ll pounds (109 pounds): 'I could not lie in the bath as my bones were sore on the bottom of the bath. My sex drive went, and I was always feeling irritable and depressed. Now when I hear slimmer success stories – you know the kind, "I lost 6 stones and my life changed completeiy" – I remark to myself, "Yeah, I bet she's lost her sex drive as well."

Mitzy wrote to Diet Breakers:

'Fat is unsexy' is a difficult one to get into, for it's an issue over which so many women feel deeply vulnerable and unhappy. Men suffer because they have internalized prejudice against fat as well – they are aware that fat women are second division and naturally want to be seen with those from the Premier League – the thin ones.

Underneath there's a lot of very different stuff going on. I know that sexuality and eroticism aren't about skinny bodies and hip bones that stick out. When you get down to the nitty-gritty, a lot of men know this as well. Sex is about bodies, flesh, touch – real people taking delight in each other.

In the media and in films the thin gals are the only ones that have the fun. In an episode in the American television series *LA Law*, a conventionally attractive man wanted to marry a larger-than-average woman. We were led to assume he was attracted to her for her money and her status and to help him get a green card to stay in America – all seemed more plausible (apparently) than the fact that he may have fancied her.

But there is a paradox here. Being thinner does not automatically increase your sexual desirability or your sexual drive. Twenty-five years ago, when I was at the height of my dieting career, I was much more interested in 'being considered attractive'. Attracting people, knowing they fancied me, was what mattered. The last thing I wanted was to have sex with them – mess up the appearance that I'd worked so hard at and ruin my perfect image! I viewed my body as a commodity rather than a part of me.

Another correspondent, Winnie, wrote,

I am five foot four, 17 stone (226 pounds) and thirty-seven years old.

I wear tight leggings, I lift weights. I am a big sexy woman who has spent years thinking I was repulsive because I'm big. I lost my man to a twenty-year-old, but he's back now. I didn't lose him because I was big but because I didn't have confidence in myself. She had the confidence to take him. Fat is irrelevant.

Finally, there is no such thing as the perfect body, even though we are led to believe otherwise. Appreciating your body as a whole, the home you live in, a being that needs feeding and nurturing to keep going, will enable you to identify with it more clearly and meet your other needs.

Making the most of our appearance

Let's do this for us. Now we are beginning to feel better about ourselves and valuing our qualities, our abilities, our personality and our body. We are responding more to internal cues and getting in touch with our real needs. So we'll be making the most of our appearance for all the right reasons – not to fit some stereotypical body shape, not to be competing with other women, not to seek approval from strangers in the street. We'll be more our own person.

Changing the way we communicate through our body language, and the way we present ourselves through our dress and grooming, can increase our confidence and feelings of self-worth. Unlike weight loss, these can be achievable and sustainable lifestyle changes.

Body language

I'm suggesting that you start to choose your body language to give the impression you want, even though at times you may feel anxious or unconfident. Body language is the way we communicate with each other without using words.

We are all experts

Reading body language is second nature to us. We are all experts: for example, when we walk down the street we manoeuvre ourselves to avoid bumping into people. We don't stop and think about it – we see the person and, as if by instinct, know whether we shall walk to the left or the right. This happens so fast and naturally that sometimes we don't even 'notice' we have seen the other person. If our reading is wrong and we collide, we both apologize in embarrassment. We can tell the difference between a mistake and someone being deliberately awkward. Yet no words have been exchanged: we have simply read each other's body language.

We 'speak' through our bodies. Whatever situation we are in, our bodies will be reflecting our thoughts and feelings about ourselves and about the people we are with. When we do speak, the tone of our voice will often convey much more than the words themselves (more on this in Chapter 8, which deals with body language in connection with assertiveness).

This aspect of communicating is partly inherited, partly learnt through culture and socialization, and partly specifically taught – such as women sitting with their knees locked together even when wearing trousers! Some Asian and Chinese people do not make eye contact – out of respect. Other communities walk one behind the other rather than side-by-side. Arab men may hold hands – which is rarely seen amongst British men.

We'll sometimes ask a close friend, 'What's wrong?' – not because of what they've said but because they are slumped forward, sighing, with their eyes staring blankly into space. Most of the time we are not thinking about our body language, or deeply analysing that of other people – it just 'happens'. In certain situations, our awareness will sharpen: when we meet someone for the first time, for instance, we may feel awkward and notice ourselves rocking on our feet, smiling unnaturally or making jerky body movements.

Feelings and thoughts related to the diet mentality, stress levels and poor body image will all be reflected in our body language. People will respond accordingly, and it will influence our 'relationship' with them.

If we take poor body image as an example, think about how you might respond to someone who is reflecting low self-esteem through their body language. That person may not be able to look you in the eye, may be adopting a closed body posture (with their arms folded across their middle, for instance), may move clumsily and may speak weakly and hesitantly.

If you are reading this as, 'This woman doesn't really like herself and is very undemonstrative', you will respond in a number of possible ways. You may feel sorry for her and feel you have to 'jolly' her along. You may patronize her because you feel superior. Or you may just feel uncomfortable in her presence. And remember, what we feel about others is often a reflection of our own feelings and insecurities.

You remind me of . . .

In my workshops, when we are doing body language exercises I remind participants to notice when they are looking at another woman which parts of her body they focus on. I then ask them to focus on their own bodies. Very often we transfer our negative feelings on to them. For example, a woman who feels uncomfortable about her own belly size may be very aware of the size of other women's bellies.

To demonstrate how easily we can be influenced by others' body language I get the group to walk around feeling miserable and to observe each other. Then I get the group to walk around being happy. Women talk about the happiness part of the experiment being 'infectious', 'feeling light' and 'wanting to smile at others'. They talk of being 'slowed' and 'heavy' or 'pulled down' by the misery.

Later I give each participant a card on which I have written certain types of behaviour. I ask the women to act and move according to what is on their card, and get the rest of the group to look at her, guess what is written on the card and say how they respond to that particular behaviour trait. Most are remarkably accurate and very observant, spotting contradictions between verbal and non-verbal communication. This is only an exercise, of course, but it is a useful way of illustrating how good we can be at reading body language and how it can influence our relationships with other people.

Becoming aware of your body language and what you are doing with your body can help you understand yourself better. Sometimes we have no idea how other people see us, so in my workshops I ask the women to form pairs. Person A of each pair watches person B walk up and down. I ask A to be aware of which areas of B's body her attention goes to, and to notice the way B moves. I then ask A to walk alongside B and copy her walk. When she feels she's got it, B drops out and observes 'her' walk.

Controlling and changing our body language can enable us to slice through some of our defensive barriers, so that later we may make refinements to the way we walk and discuss how we feel when we move our bodies differently. You could try this exercise with a friend, or even alone. Notice how you feel and, if you practise your new walk or movements in the street, how other people respond to you.

Making space

Another aspect of body language is the way we use the space around us – a complicated but well-recognized system. We communicate through four space or distance zones:

- intimate
- personal
- social
- public

As the zones imply, the more intimate we are with a person, the less personal space we need, and the closer we allow them to come to us. Sometimes, children will come closer than the 'appropriate zones' because they are not yet operating under the formal 'rules'.

When we are feeling ashamed, timid or inhibited we draw ourselves in. When we feel relaxed and confident we tend to take up more space, creating a feeling and an impression of expansiveness.

Generally speaking, in Western society men take up more space than women – both in body size and body language. This is easily observed on public transport. Groups of women together usually operate within smaller zones, but the status rules of space still apply.

When you transgress the appropriate distance zone, for example moving from the social to the personal zone when your relationship does not justify it, the other person feels you have invaded their personal space or 'buffer zone'. If this happens to you, you have a choice: you can ignore the transgression, uncomfortably endure it or do something about it. Obviously every situation is different, so it is hard to offer guidelines. If it doesn't bother you, ignore it. But if it does bother you, don't put up with it – move!

When deciding whether or not to ignore the invasion of your space you need to consider your personal comfort and how the invasion affects your status. The invasion itself is saying that you have less status than the invader because, generally speaking, higher-status people feel comfortable invading the space of people lower down the hierarchy. It is easier to picture the boss standing over the secretary than the factory worker standing over the managing director. When a woman transgresses a man's space it can be interpreted as a come-on.

If you were trying to establish yourself as a competent manager, and a member of your team made a habit of invading your space, it could matter a great deal. You might start feeling undermined, and other colleagues would be interpreting your situation in this way too. Naturally, it would be advisable not to allow this to continue.

Be aware of how much personal space you need for your comfort. Position yourself, your furniture and other possessions to give sufficient space to enable you to feel comfortable. It is impossible to feel and look confident when you are uncomfortable.

How to use body language

- Make a point of noticing other people's body language and voice tone. What impressions are you getting?

  Note: It is a mistake to draw conclusions from any one aspect of body language. Someone folding their arms may just feel more comfortable that way. We need to take into account all aspects of communication: body language, voice tone and modulation, and verbal content.

- Heighten your awareness of your own body language, particularly in tricky or challenging situations. What messages do you think you might be conveying, and is it helping or hindering you? Ask a friend whom you can rely on to give you detailed constructive feedback on your body language.

- Catch yourself when you are communicating negative messages – e.g. poor eye contact, a shuffling walk, closed body posture – and change it! Meet people eye-to-eye (but don't

stare), walk more purposefully and open out your shoulders
and chest.
- Find a role model who uses body language to her best
  advantage and copy her, until you find your own 'natural'
  way of doing it. At first it may all feel contrived, but persevere
  – the more you practise your new body language, the more it
  will become part of the real you.

Voice power

When I'm preparing myself mentally for a 'tricky' situation I also
prepare myself physically, using deep breathing exercises and
acting out and maintaining positive body language. Doing this
actually builds my confidence – try it.

We hold a lot of our emotions and power in our voice, and I
am struck by how often women have squeaky little girl voices that
do not go with their image; Jackie Onassis, for example, had just
such a voice. On the other hand Marilyn Monroe's voice seemed
perfect for a 'sex goddess' who didn't need to be taken seriously
anyway. Compare Marilyn's voice to Lauren Bacall's. Who would
doubt that she is a woman to be taken very seriously indeed?

Deep breathing – and even just remembering to breathe (we
often forget when we are fearful) – makes a real difference to
the level, pitch and tone of our voice. Becca Herisson, a musician
and singer, was shocked at her first singing lesson at university to
be told that her voice had a nice tone but that she lacked wobble
(vibrato) and that she should 'let go, stop trying to sing like a boy
treble, and "be a woman".' She went on to say,

Despite the excuses I made, this was not due to an innate weakness
in my anatomy. It was due to the fact that I thought I was fat. Like
most women who dislike the size of their bodies, I was used to walking
around trying to hold my stomach and bottom in, in the hope of looking
thinner. If I was going to sing properly (and, more importantly, if I was
to avoid damaging my vocal cords before the age of thirty) I was going
to have to use my diaphragm and the required 'expansion' – moving
your diaphragm downwards causes your stomach, your lungs and your
ribs to move outwards in all directions. If I was going to sing well, I
was going to have to stop trying to be thin.

Fortunately for me, my teacher was patient. By the time I had finally come to terms with my eating problems and the low self-esteem that was their cause, a dramatic transformation had taken place in my singing: out of the cocoon had emerged a Madam Butterfly – with wobble, with tone, with a vastly increased range, and, at last, with a smile on her face.

If you feel your voice needs more help than just practising proper breathing, it would be worth your while taking voice workshops.

Clothes

Our personal appearance is the first thing people notice about us. Clothes, hairstyle, make-up and body language all influence people's impression of us, and they then make calculated judgements about us based on that impression.

Image expert Philippa Davies says in her book *Your Total Image* that we notice a person's characteristics in the following order:

- colouring
- gender
- age
- size
- facial expression
- eye contact
- hair
- build
- clothes
- movement

Clothes are an important way of expressing and identifying ourselves. The appearance message can often be picked up easily and correctly – for example, the corporate dress code of some organizations, or the leather outfits of a group of Harley Davidson fans, and, of course, uniforms. Suits, jeans and white coats all convey distinct messages, as do ill-fitting clothes, run-down shoes and overstuffed briefcases.

Sometimes, however, our interpretations can be wildly inaccurate or based on stereotypes. For example, not all women in Essex wear white stilettos, and not all lesbians wear Doc Martens. It is worth remembering how quickly we make assumptions about people based on appearance – so that we can avoid making stereotypes ourselves, and use our appearance to work for us, creating the impressions we want people to have. Queen Mary once wrote to the then Prince of Wales, chiding him for his choice of jacket: 'Clothes are an outward form by which people can, and in general most often do, judge the inward state of mind and feelings of that person, for this they can see while the other they cannot.'

To some extent our choice of clothes is determined by what is available at the price we can afford, though my friend, designer Sarah Leedham, says she gets exasperated with the thousands of women who deprive themselves of good clothes, promising they will buy something nice when they lose weight. Women frequently tell me they want to diet because none of their clothes will fit them. Yet I never hear women sounding concerned that none of their clothes would fit if they lost weight. When buying clothes, do you consider the colours, fabrics and textures of garments and their message and status, and consider whether this matches the message you want to convey when wearing the garment? For example, beige silk would be considered more classy than tangerine lycra.

'Image' comes from a Greek word meaning 'mirage'. Thus image means a reflection of ourselves. It's the message we give to the outside world. Every morning when we get dressed – and by the way, we never put anything on by accident – we go out there and tell the rest of the world a lot about ourselves.

Have you ever spotted someone who has got it right? She's the sort of person whom you instinctively know will get it right, whether you see her wheeling her trolley round the supermarket or dressed up for dinner at a smart London hotel. Of course, what is right for one person is not necessarily 'right' for another. You know how some women can put on a tracksuit, scrape their hair up with a pin and look like a million dollars. Put another woman in the same tracksuit and she might look as if she'd been cleaning the kitchen floor!

Image training

Your clothes need to be a natural extension of yourself – they need to honour everything about *you*. If you don't feel you have got it right, it is well worth going to a good image consultant who will work with you on how to create an 'in focus' look that tells the rest of the world exactly who you are. This should include analysis of your natural colouring, body structure and, most importantly, your personality, so that your clothes venerate everything about you. It is not enough to dress just what is visible – to get it right you need to dress what is going on inside as well.

You may well ask why is it necessary to go to an image consultant to be told how to look your best – after all, you know what you like. The question is, does it like you? When most of us look in the mirror we see only how we think and feel about ourselves, and not what's really there. Everybody, without exception, is more beautiful than they actually think they are. A good image consultant will help you bridge the gap between what you see when you look in the mirror and what the rest of the world sees when it looks at you.

An image consultant friend tells the story of a client who came to a colour analysis session never having worn lipstick before. When she was given one to try, the rest of the group gasped and immediately admired the way it accentuated her hair colour, made her eyes sparkle and caused her skin to glow with health. Her reaction? 'Oh, but it makes my teeth look yellow.' No one else in the class had noticed anything wrong with her teeth – they had seen her assets while she was busy concentrating on her so-called 'faults'.

This can be a habit which we need help to overcome, and it is a good idea to go through the experience as part of a group even if you feel self-conscious at the outset. It is often easier to be objective about someone else's appearance. Through understanding what puts another person 'in focus' we become better able to accept change in ourselves. What this particular woman couldn't help admitting was that the other people in the group all looked wonderful in the clothes colours and make-up that had been suggested for them. It gave her confidence to give *her* new look a chance.

One other important lesson that this woman needed to learn was how to accept compliments. How do you react when someone pays you a compliment? It's very easy to take a compliment and sling it back where it came from. For example: 'What a great outfit you're wearing!' Reply: 'Oh, this old thing? I've had it for ages.' Or how about: 'You have the prettiest eyes.' Reply: 'I used to have, but the lines are beginning to show.' The reply to both these compliments should be quite simply 'Thank you.' It's not always an easy thing to say – particularly if you're actually feeling dreadful at the time. Try to think of a compliment as a present. If someone gives you

a present you don't open it, say 'Yuk!' and give it back to them
– it would be the height of bad manners. Practise saying 'Thank
you' to compliments, because when you're putting your best foot
forward you are likely to receive quite a lot.

So image training isn't just about learning how to look great, it's
about learning to accept that you can look wonderful every single
day. Yes, you really can be the person people look at in the street
and then say, 'Wow, she always manages to look so good!' One of
the most important things a good image consultant can do for you
is to show you something in the mirror that maybe you have never
seen before.

With this sort of confidence you will be able to start investing
in the sort of good-quality clothes that previously you had only
dreamed of. Most of us wear about 15 per cent of our wardrobe
85 per cent of the time. It's that little clutch of clothes that
come out time and time again when we want to feel comfortable, look good and make the right impression. The other 85
per cent of our wardrobe is rubbish! They might be expensive mistakes, but they are rubbish nevertheless because we're
not wearing them and they are taking up precious cupboard
space. The image consultant's job is to reduce that sort of
wardrobe to a third, but in reality to give you three times
more to wear. Can you imagine booting out that 85 per cent
and being shown how to spend your money at the level of
the 15 per cent so that everything works at maximum? What
a beautiful wardrobe you would have. What's more, you would
adore everything in it and really enjoy the daily act of getting
dressed every morning. Here are some guidelines for investment
buying.

Buy in neutral or basic colours

When buying something expensive it's well worth sticking to the
'safe' colours such as navy, black, charcoal, grey, brown, tan,
cream, beige and so on. These colours will mix and match more
easily with the rest of your wardrobe, so that you can wear them
regularly and get your money's worth.

Insist on excellent quality

If you are going to wear it often, it's got to last.

Choose a classic design

Even if you're not naturally a classic type, clothes need to have an element of 'classic' about them so that they don't date.

Flexibility

Judge each piece of an outfit in its own right. If you're buying a suit, try the jacket on its own and say to yourself, 'If I was buying a jacket, would I buy this one?' Then try the skirt and say to yourself, 'If I was buying a skirt, would I buy this one?' If the suit has flexibility it will give you the beginning of possibly thirty outfits and be worth three times what you are going to pay for it. If it doesn't have flexibility you will have bought one outfit and it won't be worth half its ticket price.

Durability

This is different for everyone, dependent on lifestyle. Ask yourself, 'Is this garment durable for the job I need it to perform?'

Comfort

It's no good buying trousers so tight that you can't sit down in them. Don't buy uncomfortable shoes and say to yourself, 'They will give after a bit' or 'I won't be walking anywhere in these.' Don't buy something that digs in or itches (and that includes underwear). You'll wear it a couple of times, and on the third occasion you'll go to the wardrobe and think, 'Oh no, I can't be bothered with that today', and you'll just stop wearing it. Remember – clothes are only expensive if you aren't wearing them.

Your clothes should flatter you

This might sound obvious, but quite often we buy something saying to ourselves, 'This will do.' You need to know and feel you look your best in a garment for it to be the sort of thing you enjoy wearing regularly.

Consider maintenance

A pale blue suede suit is not a good investment!

You must love it

If it doesn't make you feel brilliant, don't buy it. Give yourself a new rule: if you can leave the shop without it – do!

Nice but naff . . .?

A word or two now about what you should not do. If we get it wrong we run the risk of antagonizing others through the subconscious messages we give out through our clothes. In other words, we may put up very real barriers which lessen our effective communication with others. So here's a list of things that image consultants suggest you never, ever do. You might like to consider what sort of message you receive when you see someone tripping through this minefield:

- tights or socks with sandals
- an overload of jewellery
- court shoes with bare legs
- tissues
- black tights with white shoes
- plunging necklines
- white high heels
- ankle chains
- plastic carrier bags
- multiple pierced ears
- pop socks with skirts

- visible knicker lines

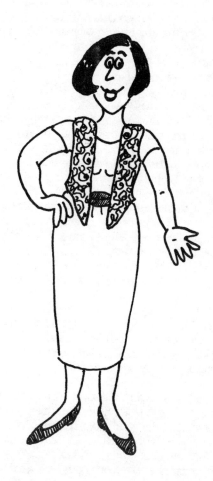

The diet breaking appearance guide

1. Always, always, always, wear clothes in which you feel comfortable and confident.
2. Choose colours that enhance your hair and skin tones. If you are not sure what suits you, save up and have your colours done by a colour analyst. She will sit you in front of a mirror

and drape you in many different shades. You will be able to see how each one works (or doesn't) for you.

3. Wear styles that suit and flatter your present size and shape. It is impossible to feel good in a crimplene tent.

4. Never buy clothes that are too small. Take the next size up and if necessary have it altered to fit you.

5. Enjoy your 'best' clothes today – don't save them, or you may end up never wearing them.

6. Swop, give away or throw out all clothes that do not fit you today. I know this may sound hard, especially if you are fond of a particular garment or it cost you a fortune. However, having clothes that don't fit you hanging there in the wardrobe can torment you and keep you wishing 'If . . .'. I put off doing this for ages, but when I did get round to it I found making the decision and putting the items in the bag was the worst bit. Once they were gone I quickly forgot them.

7. It is hard to look or feel assertive and confident in six-inch heels. They also wreck your back and feet, affect your breathing and stop you running from danger. Save them for parties.

8. Your hair is your crowning glory. Keep it clean and in good condition. Have it cut by a good hairdresser every six to eight weeks in a style that you can manage yourself between visits to the salon.

9. Keep your hands well moisturized and manicured – whether you wear your nails long or short (all the same length, please!). Remove chipped nail polish immediately.

10. If you like to wear make-up but don't feel confident applying it, or feel it isn't working for you, consider having a make-up lesson.

11. Keep your skin clean, regularly exfoliated and always well moisturized. It will look and be healthier and protected from the drying effects of wind, cold and sun.

12. Stand evenly on both feet – it will help you breathe better as well as look and feel more confident.

13. Allow your facial expressions to match what you are saying. No apologetic or ghost smiles.

14. Make good eye contact when you speak to people. Don't try to outstare them aggressively or to be demurely shy like Princess Di used to be. Think what kind of message it conveys; it might have worked for Diana when her role was 'pretty princess', but it does not work for diet breaking women who want to be taken seriously. I notice Di has recently changed this aspect of her body language.

15. Avoid drawing imaginary pictures in the air with your finger when you are describing things. It gives the impression that you don't know – and gives people the excuse to dismiss what you are saying.
16. Don't play, fiddle, suck or flick your hair – it looks daft and many men think it is a come-on. If you don't mean it to be, you may end up with unwanted attention.

The dieter's worry is of losing control and of the drastic consequences – including not being attractive enough. Improving our body image and the way we present ourselves are areas that are within our power to influence positively, and will give us feelings of personal power. Unlike the goal of weight loss, these changes are sustainable and we eliminate the fear factor of 'What will happen if . . .'. We start from a basis of self-acceptance and enhancement rather than criticism and self-loathing, so we are working with our body rather than fighting against it.

8

Take the 'A' Train – and Influence Your World

Somewhere over the rainbow . . .

It is a lamentable fact that the reason many women diet is because they are unhappy. Perhaps they are lonely or feel they are not successful enough, or are shy or insecure. Somewhere along the journey we have picked up and swallowed the myth that being slim will provide the key to a magic wonderland where we will have the gifts of confidence, success and beauty. We will be desirable and sexy, the centre of attention, the life of any party, the fixer of any problem.

From time to time, perhaps, you had nagging doubts about whether everything would indeed miraculously fall into place. However, since most other women believed in it too, you may have thought you were the only person for whom the magic wasn't working. I hope by now you will have recognized that it is only a myth.

It isn't realistic to expect life to be like one long glossy advertisement, where all our needs are met and there is never a nasty thought or problem in sight. We create our own reality, and for the majority of us sometimes it's wonderland and sometimes it feels more like hell. The not-so-good times can provide opportunities for us to discover more about ourselves, so that we can learn from our experiences and move on. By dealing with the real issues that are facing us, and by enjoying our successes, we do gain confidence. I went to an exhibition of children's art and the title of one child's creation summed it up nicely: *No Rain, no Rainbow*.

Individually and collectively we can change the agenda to ensure that all women and girls have a better way of living – starting with you! By finding ways to look after and nurture yourself you will feel better about yourself, and then you can reach out to influence what is happening in the wider community.

We did not wake up one morning with a sudden desire to be two sizes smaller, nor did we develop dissatisfaction with our bodies out of thin air. Our need to be constantly dieting is a symptom of our society and its present values; a healthy person flourishes in a healthy society. Because our thin bodies have become the yardstick with which society measures virtue, we have, in effect, been appointed the guardians of virtue for our culture.

It's a heavy-duty responsibility, for which we receive no real advantages or reward. The real benefit is that we are saved from the punishment that society imposes on lunatics, heretics, anarchists and women who refuse to do as they are told. I guess some people may see us as all of these.

It is exciting to realize that we diet breakers are on the threshold of changing society, and that we can have a direct impact on making things more like we want them to be – for ourselves and for others. I know some people believe the change is happening anyway – as people in general become more aware of their spiritual selves and get in tune with their physical bodies, so we are evolving into a non-dieting society in which we will nurture ourselves appropriately on all levels.

Taking the steps necessary to bring ourselves back to good health and self-respect is essential. However, to be really successful we need to influence our society so that the girls and women who follow us can be safeguarded from the tyranny of thinness and can be assured of a place on the 'A' train! So this chapter is about making change for the better – for ourselves, for others and for society.

Changing ourselves part 1: goal setting

I hope you will have gained from this book lots of ideas about changes you want to make within yourself, in others and in the outside world. If you are already incorporating some of them into your life, remember the diet breaking process in Chapter 4 which prepares you for the possible negative feelings of denial, anger and depression which may follow the initial euphoria of diet breaking. We can work towards a better way of living by establishing measures of success for ourselves which are in no way related to thinness or body 'perfection'.

Knowing what you want to achieve and how it will benefit you, talking about it to others who will listen and support you, and then working out a plan for yourself will give you a greater chance of succeeding. This life of ours is not a dress rehearsal – this is it! Don't squander it. I look on how I spend my time as an investment of me in the various areas of my life, and ask myself what it's doing for me in terms of pay-offs. And I don't necessarily mean money. Receiving a salary or wage and having the ability to be secure and enjoy life is an obvious pay-off, but I also consider what return I'm getting on my investment in other ways.

Nurturing and sustaining my friendships, for example, gives me feelings of love, appreciation and a sense of belonging, together with the knowledge that I can call on my friends when I need support or encouragement. Through starting and developing the Diet Breakers campaign I have become a 'new' person. I have become more knowledgeable about the way the dieting industry works; I know more about health and nutrition; my eyes have been opened to the appalling prejudice with which fat people are regarded; I have developed skills in producing a magazine and writing articles; I have become more aware of my own attitude to dieting and body image; I have increased my self-esteem; and I have enjoyed the positive acknowledgements and esteem of others. And, last but not least, I feel I am maximizing my abilities and striving to reach my full potential, which I find is an incredibly powerful motivator.

This goal-setting exercise will help you define what you want to do to develop yourself and identify the steps you need to take to get you there. You will need your journal or a large sheet of paper to write your ideas down. Remember, the journey (process) can be as rewarding as arriving at your destination (achieving your goals).

1. Write down your vision of how you want to be

You might start by saying something like 'I want to free myself from the diet mentality', or 'I want to end my obsession of dissatisfaction with my body.'

Move from those statements to something which is positive and forward-looking. Visualize what you would 'look like' if these were achieved. You may want to sit comfortably and undisturbed and close your eyes to do this.

Your vision could look something like this. Imagine a woman who stands, walks and moves in a manner which exudes confidence, wearing clothes that enhance her beauty and style. She has fully integrated her body into her persona, giving the impression that she is at home in her body, she 'owns' it and loves it. She has put food in its rightful place and has found other ways of meeting her emotional needs. She is her own person, who values her unique qualities and strives to notice and appreciate the individual qualities of others. She is working to achieve a range of goals in her life which are exciting, challenging and achievable.

2. Write down the ways in which an 'outsider' will notice the difference in you – what will be the 'evidence' that you have changed?

As an example, you may have done things that you have never done before or not done for a very long time – twirled around a dance floor with lots of people looking at you, or developed new friendships which are separate from your roles of mother, daughter, wife, lover and so on.

3. How long will it take you – what is a realistic time frame for you to achieve the new you?

Choose a completion date that is not so soon that you will fail and not so far in the future that it won't be challenging.

4. What will you have to stop doing in order to do the activities which will take you to your destination?

For instance, my partner will need to prepare his/her own meal on two evenings a week to give me the extra time I need.

5. Choosing your goals

A. Write down everything in your head (brainstorm) that you will have to do to achieve your vision

At this stage go for quantity, not quality. Don't be analytical – go even for the seemingly crazy ideas. The things you need to do may include 'jobs' like buying a book, going on a course or starting a journal. They will include changes you want to make within yourself, such as saying 'no' more often, and they will include interaction with other people, like plucking up courage to talk with your mother about your decision to stop dieting.

This is an example of how such a list might look:

Stop dieting at once
Chuck out bathroom scales
Chuck out clothes that I'll never get into
Burn all my diet books
Don't get involved in facile conversations about weight
Eat three meals a day
Find a physical activity that I will enjoy
Stop buying magazines that over-promote dieting and slenderness
Buy a journal and write something in it every day
Reward myself when I have achieved something that was difficult
Increase my confidence
Start loving my body
Buy a full-length mirror
Start going to dance/movement classes
More research needed to get the right class for me
Get a new job
Ditch my boyfriend – maybe not, tell him where I'm at, and give him a chance to change his attitude
Say 'no' more often
Overcome my shyness when meeting new people
Stop giving my personal power away
Join a group
Draw up book list
Find a course to go on
Spend more time with my friend – she really is on my wavelength
Save up to see an image/colour consultant
Do more things to nourish myself spiritually

Write out affirmations and stick them on the walls
Positive images of women of all sizes
Be more appreciative of the women I meet – tell them!
Stop seeking approval of any Tom, Dick . . .
Catch myself comfort eating and work out an alternative response
Arrange to have some counselling or psychotherapy
Stop trying to be perfect
Let go once in a while – yippee!
Stop feeling guilty all the bloody time
Get out of bed in the morning with a positive attitude
Buy some new clothes
Have a walk every day
Go out more – make the effort
Organize a holiday, a day out, a special treat that I've been
denying myself
I've always wanted to learn a new skill – go to evening class

B. Sleep on it

When you have written down everything you can think of, don't
worry if your list seems enormous. It's good to have a lot to choose
from. Take one last look at the list and add anything else that comes
to mind. Then sleep on it. Next day, look at your list again and add
any more items that have come to mind overnight.

C. Prioritize

You can't do it all at once. Identify two or three long-term goals
– ones that will take six months or more to achieve – that, if you
worked on them, you believe would give you real and beneficial
change. For example, if you chose 'building my confidence', put
an asterisk against all the things on your list that are relevant to
that goal. Breaking down a seemingly big and complex objective
into smaller elements helps you to get going and make gradual but
real progress. Devise a grid like the one shown on p 177, with a
list of tasks and their start and completion dates.

   From your list there may also be a number of short-term goals
that are easily achievable and will give you a quick or easy pay-off.
For example, buying yourself some new clothes or taking out a
magazine subscription, becoming a member of Diet Breakers
and so on.

D. Schedule and plan

Start booking items from the grid into your diary and journal as a way of ensuring that you will stick to your goals. Acknowledge that you are making progress by marking with a tick or star when you complete one of your tasks. It's good to flip back in the diary and see a constellation of gold stars, for instance – they remind us of how far we have travelled.

Tips:

- Don't be over-ambitious: work at a pace that is comfortable for you so as to avoid unnecessary disappointments.
- Don't over-schedule your diary: leave enough time and space to cope with everyday hassles and crises that crop up.
- Adopt a flexible approach: as circumstances change, you may want to change goals too.
- Look at your main goals every day and ask yourself two questions: (1) given the way I am spending my time, am I getting what I want? and (2) what am I doing today to progress my goals?
- Don't be obsessive: take a relaxed, step-by-step approach.

Changing ourselves part 2: assertiveness

This next section is still about changing ourselves as well as influencing our world. Being more assertive will enable you to deal with situations more effectively, which will help increase your confidence and self-esteem, which in turn will bring you greater respect from others.

Let's start with the Diet Breakers' Bill of Rights, which was developed by Roz Juma and myself. Bodyism and the tyranny of thinness cause us confusion, so the purpose of this Bill is to remind us that we do have rights, and to make us realize what they are.

You will see that some of the items are rights that only you can give yourself: numbers 1, 2, 7, 14 and 15 probably fall into this category. However, as you gain confidence and grant yourself these rights, so your expectation of being treated fairly will impact on others. This will further increase your confidence and give you the strength to insist on your rights from people and organizations who are letting you down.

The Diet Queen

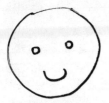   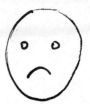

I'm a lot more
attractive
than you

The Diet Victim

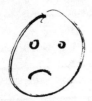

You're a lot
more attractive
than me

The Diet Club Member

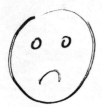

If only we
were more
attractive

The Diet Manipulator

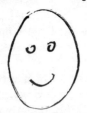   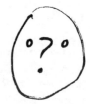

You look nice –
have you lost/
gained weight

The Diet Breaking Woman

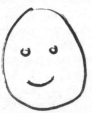   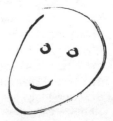

I'm learning to accept
my beauty and I can
appreciate yours too

I have noticed that when I afford myself my basic rights I feel proud and self-respecting, and when I don't I feel sad because I let myself down. So the very act of standing up for yourself can contribute to your feeling stronger as well as earning you better treatment from others.

Look at the list and think about what the Bill of Rights means for you. Make a mental note (or write one in your journal) of which rights you are currently granting yourself and which ones you need to be working on.

The Diet Breakers' Bill of Rights

1. I have the right to be treated with respect.
2. I have the right to challenge bodyism and sizeism alongside racism, sexism and ageism.
3. I have the right to be considered on the merits of who I am, not who society perceives me to be.
4. I have the right to feel and look good.
5. I have the right to expect a full range of affordable, attractive clothes – correctly labelled.
6. I have the right to be seen by the media and reflected as part of society on TV and in magazines and newspapers.
7. I have the right to be happy and healthy and to enjoy life to the full.
8. I have the right to compete for job opportunities based on my skills and abilities.
9. I have the right to enjoy and exercise my body.
10. I have the right to access public services and transport.
11. I have the right to expect full, professional, unbiased and appropriate health care.
12. I have the right to be considered as a potential foster/adoptive parent on my merits and suitability – not my appearance.
13. I have the right to eat and enjoy food.
14. I have the right to say 'yes' and 'no' – without feeling guilty.
15. I have the right to be me.

Let's start with something positive. Think of situations where you usually give yourself your rights, and what the benefits are to your feelings and the situation.

Are there some rights that you have difficulty giving yourself? I am not talking here about those that you want from others – for the moment concentrate on those that you can give to yourself. Are you prepared to accept your rights, or are you holding yourself back at all?

If you are finding it hard to give yourself rights, think about how you are holding yourself back and start working towards them today.

1. Make three photocopies of the Bill of Rights.
2. Put one on your wall at home.
3. Put one on your wall at work, or carry it in your bag, to remind you of your rights should you forget them.
4. Show the third copy to a friend and discuss the various aspects with her/him.

What assertiveness really means

Naturally, we diet breaking women are assertive women. We start from the basis that all women and men deserve respect. diet breaking women are not goddesses: we do not have to like everyone, or demand that everyone likes us. We merely start off by believing that, regardless of our abilities, size, weight, looks, attractiveness and so on, we are all of value, we all have something to contribute and we all have something to learn.

Dieting can prevent us from being assertive, because the very essence of the diet game is to pollute our thinking, which contaminates our relationships with ourselves and other women along the lines of the illustration on p 174.

Being assertive is essential if you are going to break out of the vicious diet trap. Assertiveness is a philosophy, a way of life, that will stand you in good stead in all areas of your life, not just in the matter of dieting. Being assertive means respecting ourselves and taking responsibility for ourselves, our actions and the consequences. When we are assertive we communicate our needs, wants, feelings, opinions and beliefs in direct, honest and appropriate ways. We recognize our rights and those of others. Dieting and dissatisfaction with our body diverts us from getting our needs satisfied in appropriate and nourishing ways.

The slimming industry maintains that women are being assertive when they choose to diet. This suggestion is as facile as suggesting that the people in Bosnia are assertive when they collect the food

PERSONAL GOAL: Building my confidence	Start date	Completion date
Membership subscription to Diet Breakers		
Books on aasertiveness/women's relationship with food/body image Visit book shop/library Decide when my best time for reading is (what will I have to give up?)		

Assertiveness training course
 	
Gather information first: libary
                                         bookshop
                                         (friend)
Communicate decision to my partner
Sort out finances
Book course		

Use my journal to record my achievements, small and large		
Get my support systems organized Who are they/how do they support me? List what kind of support I want from them Rehearse asking them for support Plan a strategy		
My difficult social/'family' situations Make a list from the least to the most fearful Address my blockages – what makes them fearful? Talk them over with (my friend on support network) to assess risk factors and work out strategies Clarify the outcomes I want Choose ones that are important for me to progress		
Personal presentation Buy that outfit I knew I wanted but was too shy to wear Investigate cost, availability of image/colour consultant Make a decision		
Therapist Gather information from (my friend) Look for recommendation (check whether they are in the diet mentality themselves) Think through whether this is really what I want Make a decision		

distributed by the aid services. As the DB survey showed, the decision to diet has more to do with social trends and circumstances – which, of course, the dieting, food and fashion industries have spent millions of pounds and dollars shaping.

The whole point of dieting means we are abiding by other people's rules. By definition, we diet breaking women make our own rules that are fair and enriching – to ourselves and others. It isn't always appropriate to be assertive. For example, there may be times when you think that the pay-off may not be worth the effort. Or perhaps you feel tired. So don't make being assertive a rod for your own back, so that you feel you have to be assertive or you will be 'letting the side down'. The only person who can decide if an event or situation is important to you is you. In an average day there will be a myriad of opportunities for you to be assertive. The key is to respond in a way that will help you, without demeaning or punishing other people.

The put-downs

Jo Ind, women's editor of the *Birmingham Post* and author of that enjoyable and enlightening book, *Fat is a Spiritual Issue*, came to speak at the 1994 International No Diet Day Rally. She told us about her train journey down to London from Birmingham. She was hungry and went to the buffet car to get something to eat. When she had made her selection of a large coffee and small bar of chocolate, the man serving said, 'Tut, tut . . . wicked!'

Given the number of women he serves each day, it is reasonable to suppose he has made this comment more than once. Now, Jo had the choice of whether to pick up the man's point or ignore it. This is how the conversation continued.

Jo: 'Why wicked?'
Man: 'Er . . . umm . . .'
Jo: 'It's not wicked – it's what I want.'

Man looks embarrassed and attempts to smile.

Jo: 'Chocolate itself is not wicked. The surest way to make eating an emotional issue is to label some food as "OK" and other food as "wicked".'

Let's examine what was going on here, and identify Jo's assertive reply. The man is in the diet mentality (thinking foods are either good or bad). He feels he has a right to comment on a woman's food choices. Can you imagine him saying the same to another man? I can't. Jo put it back to him by asking a question, and when he struggled to come back with a reply she clearly refuted his comment and assumption, asserting her right to make her own food choices without being made to feel guilty.

Laura wrote, 'My boyfriend once said he couldn't fancy anyone who was fat. When I asked how he'd feel if I put on weight he said he'd still love me, but wouldn't fancy me. He is very conscious of his own weight and shape too.' Laura's boyfriend's comment is a good example of the tyranny. Once expressed, a remark can cut deeply into your psyche, and you can be held hostage ever after.

Peggy's sister, for instance, had said something similar nearly thirty years earlier, and for years she worried.

About fifteen years passed before I eventually decided to confront her about it. I turned to my inner directory – that place where I store up everything people say or do that hurts me – and I repeated what she had said all those years before.

'Did I say that?'

'Yes.'

'When was that?'

'August 1968, when we were on holiday in Scarborough.'

'Oh, for God's sake, Peg, I was twenty-one. I didn't know any better. Of course I don't feel like that now!' and she gave me a hug.

Disbelieving, I looked at her closely. Could I trust her? Was she telling the truth, or was she just saying it?

Then she said, 'I am shocked that you think I could feel like that for all these years.'

This conversation helped both of us. At last I was free to talk about my feelings and fears, and Dulcie understands me more too.

I would urge Laura to talk to her boyfriend about his statement. Check out whether it still holds true for him. Perhaps he too has changed his mind now. He probably doesn't know what effect this statement has had on her. If he has changed his values, then the problem is solved. If he still holds this view, at least he will be aware of the pressure he is putting on Laura. Gradually, as Laura grows more confident and assertive, she will see that the problem is her boyfriend's not hers – and, hopefully, as this happens she will leave it to him to deal with. In other words, he must take responsibility for himself.

Assertiveness exercise

The following exercise can be useful in many situations, from negotiations with colleagues and friends to those that are more emotionally charged, like Laura's. When we're being assertive we are looking for a win-win situation. The more specific we are, the greater chance we have of achieving a successful outcome. Before you begin, think through the following:

- What you are feeling
- What you would like to come from the negotiation
- What would be an assertive outcome

Of course, the outcome we would like may not be assertive, in which case you may have to give a little. Think it through, take a deep breath to help you stay calm and to strengthen your voice, and then proceed:

Stage 1

When you . . . (describe behaviour)   By describing the behaviour you enable the listener to understand what you mean.

Stage 2

I feel . . .   In saying how you feel, you avoid blaming the other person. If you start blaming, they will become aggressive or defensive.

Stage 3

I would like/prefer/want . . .   Honestly declaring your preference encourages the listener to be honest too, and creates a stronger possibility of reaching an agreed decision or compromise.

If at Stage 3 you are not able to reach agreement, you will need to choose your next step, for example:

Stage 4

| **In that case . . .** | I would like to think about things for a couple of days. I want you to know I am not happy about this. I would like you to read Diet Breaking/another book, to help you understand my feelings and position. I would like us to have couples' therapy. |

Your route at Stage 4 will depend on the situation, on your relationship with the person, on whether you feel it is worth investing your time and emotions, and on what consequences you wish to take. Don't make empty threats – they are not assertive and they don't work.

Choosing techniques

In most situations you have a choice of assertive techniques, which is why thinking ahead to what you would like to get from the situation is essential. For example, Barbara wrote: 'A colleague of mine said I was just thin enough to be her friend, otherwise I would have been too fat.'

Barbara has a choice of techniques, depending on what she wants to get from the situation. She could use the above technique, or the technique of enquiry in which she asks for information before giving her response: 'How does my size affect you?' Or she could be completely up front and say, 'I find your comment offensive and hurtful', which is what Sadia said to her colleagues who were making fun of Sarah Ferguson for putting on weight. Her colleagues went quiet and stopped the conversation. Sadia put her head down and carried on working. A few hours later one of her colleagues had thought it through and apologised. This gave Sadia the opportunity to explain her feelings further and thus recruit an ally. This would not have happened if she had not taken the risk to honour her feelings and speak out.

Often our tone of voice and our body language, rather than our words, determines whether we are being assertive, aggressive or passive. Experts in the study of body language believe around 38 per cent of the message is received from the tone of voice, compared with just 7 per cent from the actual words. The remaining 55 per cent is received through our body language. We want our non-verbal communication to match the content of what we are saying, so that we don't give mixed messages.

If Sadia had shrugged her shoulders or giggled at the end of what she said, she might not have been taken seriously. Our voice needs to be calm, evenly paced, and with no intonation that would suggest hostility or sarcasm. Our body language should be open, in other words shoulders back, arms resting in a comfortable position, preferably not crossed, and, whether we are standing or sitting, we should not be fidgeting or rocking. Making eye contact with the other person in a friendly way will ensure that you both feel 'connected' to each other and the conversation.

Timing, too, can make all the difference. It is virtually impossible to be assertive when you are reeling with anger or lacerated with pain.

Have you ever felt you have over-responded to a situation? Perhaps a person has said or done something that in itself does not seem particularly significant, and yet it affects you a lot. You go 'over the top' or withdraw into your shell. The transaction or situation may have reminded you of a past experience, either consciously or subconsciously, and you react as you did to the old situation rather than to what is happening now. So remember to choose a time that suits you and when the other person will be able to hear your message.

When someone throws you a ball, you do not have to catch it. The same goes for a rude or hurtful remark. Given prac- tice, you can step aside and let such remarks fly past you, or you can catch them and throw them back by asking a ques- tion. With this technique, patronizing remarks or back-handed compliments can be adroitly handled. Pauline heard this one: 'Not many fat people are brave enough to wear dungarees.' Reply: 'Not brave, but free to wear whatever I choose. Do

you have a problem with a woman my size wearing dungarees?'

If the person making such a remark is close or important to you,
you could risk being assertively honest: 'I am really hurt by your
comment.' Notice here you are owning the feeling, not blaming
the other person.

Turning your emotions to advantage

How do you decide whether being assertive is appropriate or worth
your time and effort? Consider these aspects of the situation:

- How important is the person to me?
- How important is this event?
- What impact or repercussions will there be if (a) I ignore it,
  or (b) I handle it assertively?

There will undoubtedly be occasions when you won't want to be
assertive. Janet said, 'I hate comments such as "Don't eat that, it'll
make you get fat", or "You shouldn't be eating that." I usually
meet them with "Mind your own business." I don't like people
telling me I should be thinner, or not, for that matter.' But not
everyone is like Janet.

As a child, when I got upset at other children calling me names,
my dad would say, 'That's nothing. Don't let a silly little thing
like that upset you.' I knew he meant well – perhaps he couldn't
bear to see me upset or hurt – but the consequence was that I
became confused about my feelings. So I swallowed my hurt and
learned that in my family it was more acceptable to express anger
than hurt.

It took years before I realized that tears and anger may be
the flip side of the same coin. Some people show anger when
underneath they really feel like crying. Others may cry and be
masking their anger. A third group may not be sure quite what they
are feeling. If you are feeling angry, hurt or confused about dieting
and the tyranny of thinness, honour your feelings as legitimate and
consider how you can direct them to achieve positive outcomes for
yourself and others. For example, anger at an advertisement can be
directed, in an assertive way, to the appropriate organization. You
are making your feelings known and, even if you don't immediately

get the changes you are wanting, you will have unloaded some of your anger in a positive way.

A friend of mine says when she was growing up she never saw her parents shout or row. They rarely hugged or kissed – everything was very even, well-mannered and 'nice'. She says she became confused and guilty about her feelings, but once she learned to express her anger, to show her emotions and to be assertive, she felt wonderfully liberated.

Putting it into practice

Let's look at some more real life situations:

Situation

Penny's friend had told her, 'You're too pretty to be so big.'

Analysis

This is a back-handed compliment: it appears to be a compliment but in fact it is a put-down.

- There is an assumption that it is OK to make such comments.
- It objectifies women.

Intention and effect

The friend may say, 'I didn't mean that' or 'That wasn't my intention.' But as adults we need to take responsibility for our comments and behaviour.

Penny's choice

- To *challenge* the comment (aggressive)
- To laugh (passive)
- To ignore it (passive)
- To deal with it (assertive)

In making her decision Penny has to consider the consequences of the various options open to her.

Consequences of the choices

- *Aggressive challenge*: The friend may become defensive and be unable to hear Penny's justified objections. *Outcome*: unsatisfactory to both parties.
- *Laughing*: May endear Penny to her friend but it would also encourage more such 'jokes'. *Outcome*: Penny is demeaned.
- *Ignoring*: Penny would appear to be condoning the comment because her friend would be unaware of her true feelings. *Outcome*: problem remains.
- *Dealing with the situation assertively*: Enables Penny to explain her feelings about the remark and why she finds it offensive. *Outcome*: the friend is more able to hear Penny's view, and can grasp the opportunity to review her behaviour. Possibly greater mutual respect has been engendered.

Coping assertively

There are a number of assertive ways of dealing with a remark like this, depending on the circumstances and timing. According to the outcome you are looking for and the investment you want to make, you may decide to talk to your friend when you are alone and explain why you think such comments are unacceptable. This approach gives you time to calm your feelings and plan what you are going to say and, importantly, means your friend does not have to 'lose face' in front of other people. Of course, in choosing a strategy you must weigh up whether or not your standing will be affected by leaving the matter until later.

Assertive statement: 'I am pretty and I am big.'

Assertive enquiry: 'What do you mean?' or 'Is that a compliment?'

Assertive disclosure: 'I am offended (and hurt – optional) when you say that, because it sounds like a compliment when in fact it's an insult.'

Assertive statement and request: 'My appearance is not up for discussion, so I'd appreciate you keeping your opinions to yourself.'

Quick responses sometimes come in handy, so it's useful to keep a few up your sleeve: 'Thank you', 'Yes, more to love', 'Don't I look great', 'Not just a pretty face' or 'and I've got brains too'.

Speaking up for yourself

Do you ever hear people talking about a third person and get the feeling that their comments are meant for you? Or perhaps the comments are not meant for you but none the less affect you? What do you do in such circumstances? Do you, through lack of assertiveness, put up with it and stay silent, fearful that the other people involved would otherwise think you were over-reacting or hypersensitive?

Speaking up for yourself is a good way of valuing yourself and letting people know how their behaviour impacts on others. Remember, if we don't actually speak up, we miss the opportunity to help people to learn and change. Also, if we don't speak up we give people an excuse for not changing ('Oh, I didn't realize, I had no idea you felt like that . . .').

One Diet Breakers' supporter told me that a couple of her thin friends were saying how awful it was that they were getting fat. Monica said to her friends, 'How do you think I feel listening to you? You're both size 12, and you are saying how awful it is to be fat. What are you saying about me at size 18? Are you saying I'm awful?'

There was some nervous protestations, 'Oh no, of course not, and anyway, we don't think of you as fat.' But the situation created an opportunity for them to open up dialogue about size oppression and bodyism, and it has helped her two friends to feel better about themselves too.

Talking about size, I get irritated when I'm speaking to journalists over the phone and suddenly they say, 'What size are you?' I used to ask them, 'What relevance does my size have?' Now I say, 'I'm my size', and leave it at that. It's a useful response to have up your sleeve.

In the short term it is often easy to let comments go, but you may be left with an uneasy feeling if you say nothing, particularly in situations where people are meddling where they have no right.

Situation

Gerty was getting married for the second time. Her husband-to-be told her his grown-up children thought she was too fat to be his wife. Gerty felt hurt that the stepchildren should be so unkind and let down by Ralph for (apparently) not publicly supporting her.

Analysis

Any prejudice can be used as a scapegoat for other concerns. People's problem with size or appearance has more to do with their own problems. Speculating, we might wonder whether it has to do with acquiring a stepmother. Or perhaps they fear their father's choice will be seen as a reflection on them: in other words, they fear they will be judged negatively by others, based on their stepmother's size.

I can relate to Gerty's stepchildren. When I was a child I spent my summer holidays with my mother and grandmother in Brighton. Every year we would sit on the stony beach eating sandwiches and ice cream, and every year my grandmother would sit with a bath towel wrapped round her head and shoulders. If the weather was sunny she would say it was to keep the sun off her face, and if it wasn't sunny she said it was to keep the wind from blowing her hair. I found her behaviour most embarrassing, and I hated her making 'us' look daft.

As the years passed I got to see it was her that was 'looking daft', not me. Now, when I see old pictures of my grandmother walking along the street looking like a cross between an Arab woman and a gypsy, I admire her strength and eccentricity.

Naturally Gerty feels hurt by the comments of her new stepchildren. But it is essential for her to hang on to the belief that it is their problem, not hers. These stepchildren are adults and must find their own way to self-acceptance – without demeaning Gerty. She has the choice of whether or not to broach the subject with the stepchildren. For my part I believe it is more important that she talks it over with her husband, to get him on her side and insist on his loyalty and support.

Assertiveness in the face of health tyrants

A year or so back I was on holiday and contracted a low-grade infection. I went to a local health centre where I received excellent treatment – apart from one small thing. I was routinely weighed.

When I asked the nurse why she wanted to weigh me, she said, 'It is this health centre's policy to weigh all patients. It's good health care practice.' This all sounds very good, but I got to thinking how useless it was to weigh me anyway – first, my weight had no bearing on my infection, and secondly, she didn't measure my height as well. What did the information tell the doctor? I wondered. I expressed these views to the nurse and doctor. Surprisingly, both agreed and said nobody had questioned it before.

An excellent way for women to begin getting health care professionals to consider their views is to refuse to be weighed. Of course there are times when it is necessary, for example during pregnancy or when monitoring drugs and medications. Often we are weighed or given weight-loss lectures irrespective of the illness for which we have requested professional help. I would like all health professionals to consider why they want to weigh patients. The knowledge that they will be weighed can prevent some women from getting the health treatment they need because of the embarrassment or guilt they are made to feel. Seeing health only in terms of size and weight may have more to do with the health provider's attitudes than it does with our health.

In America, activists are beginning to take a stand over the medical care they receive. Women are complaining about negative attitudes and treatments and are questioning certain assumptions from health providers – such as automatically weighing patients or prescribing diets. Fat people are demanding appropriate equipment and facilities, too, such as gowns that fit. Such action, of course, takes courage, and when we are unwell we don't always feel up to taking a stand even though the quality of care and attention can make all the difference to our recovery. If you are not satisfied with your health treatment, do something about it when you feel able.

Remember: it is not always necessary to be weighed. If you don't want to be weighed, assert your right not to be. Consent to treatment rests with the patient – and you are the patient, not the patsy.

Scenario 1

Ivy goes to the health centre with a vaginal infection. To ascertain appointment priority, patients are first referred to the reception nurse. Ivy explains what is wrong and is directed to a small room, asked to remove her tights and pants and told that someone will be with her shortly. The nurse comes in, takes her blood pressure, weighs her, writes down the information and leaves. A few minutes later the doctor comes in, asks a few questions, writes out a prescription and directs her down the corridor to the pharmacist. Ivy leaves the health centre with her medication.

Scenario 2

As above, until the nurse comes into the room to take Ivy's blood pressure and weigh her. Ivy tells the nurse she does not want to be weighed. The nurse asks, 'Why?' Ivy says her weight is not relevant to the vaginal infection or to the medication she needs. The nurse goes out to speak to the doctor. The doctor returns with the nurse. Ivy confirms that she doesn't wish to be weighed. The nurse leaves. The doctor asks, 'Why?' Ivy gives the same reasons to the doctor as she did to the nurse and goes on to explain that many women do not feel comfortable about seeking health treatment because they fear being lectured and weighed. Ivy explains that she is part of the campaign to challenge the tyranny of thinness. The doctor listens closely, and asks for information on the campaign. Two months later a notice goes up in the waiting room:

THIS PRACTICE RESPECTS THE RIGHT OF ALL PATIENTS TO CHOOSE WHETHER OR NOT TO BE WEIGHED. PATIENTS ARE WEIGHED ONLY AFTER DISCUSSION AND WHEN BOTH PARTIES AGREE THE INFORMATION WILL CONTRIBUTE TO THE PATIENT'S TREATMENT.

As I have said elsewhere in this book, the tyranny affects us all, whatever our weight. Automatic weigh-ins are something we can all challenge.

No to bitchiness

We are led to believe that bitching about others is the main feature of women's conversations, which of course is sexist rubbish. Not all women talking together are bitches, but that is not to deny it goes on – and not just with women! I have found that when I don't take part in 'bitchy' discussions people soon decide I am not eligible for the 'Gossip Club'. It doesn't stop the gossip, but it keeps me out of it.

Another way to handle these kinds of conversations is to open up dialogue, for example:

Friend: 'Look at her – what does she look like? She's put on weight recently.'

You: 'How does what she looks like affect you?' or 'I really value our friendship. However, I feel uncomfortable when you run so-and-so down because of her weight/clothes/etc.'

Friend: 'Why?'

You: 'I don't think it's productive. It encourages us to value each other on what we look like rather than on what we have to offer. I like to keep a positive frame of mind.'

And if you wanted to explain further . . .

'This kind of conversation hooks into my insecurities about body image. In my experience I find these types of conversations are not at all empowering – we only feel better than the person we are putting down.'

Learning to be assertive with nearest and dearest

Christine, the woman I met on the train to Newcastle, is not the only woman to tell me about husbands or partners putting pressure on them because of their appearance. Holly told me her husband has a habit of making disparaging remarks about her size, shape or choice of clothes. She said, 'He seems to do it mostly when I get something new, or when I'm just going out of the door.'

When you are starting a new relationship you are in a good position to make it clear that your personal appearance is not up for debate. Persecutors have a gift for sniffing out victims, so if this is their bag they will quickly get the message that you are not prepared to be persecuted by them, and will leave you alone.

If your partner, parents or friends do this sort of thing to you, it is important for you to make sure you are not colluding. Don't open up a dialogue about your appearance. Don't ask for this person's opinion on how you look or ask them whether you look all right. If you do, you are giving them an invitation to wade in with criticism – and, yes, they always seem to pick the perfect moment to burst your bubble. At some stage you will need to negotiate with the person, letting them know that things are changing and that you want them to stop this criticism.

Being assertive with our nearest and dearest is often the hardest area of all, so practise with a friend, or rehearse what you are going to say on the bus, or as you drive to work. When you have got the words right, and you feel strong within yourself, you might want to say something along these lines:

You: 'We have got into a situation where you habitually criticize my appearance, and I appreciate that I have played a part too by not stopping you. However, I want you to stop criticizing me now (optional: because I find it hurtful and upsetting).'

Other person: 'Oh, don't be so touchy.'

You: 'I'm not being touchy. I'm just telling you that I don't want you to be rude about my appearance.'

Other person: 'Well, you always ask me what I think,' or 'Well, you don't look as good as you used to' etc.

You: 'I know what I look like, and I want you to stop criticizing me.'

Avoid getting sidetracked into irrelevancies or put-downs such as your dress sense, and don't expect this person to agree instantly and be matey-matey with you. Allow him or her to mull over what you have said, so resist giving lots of examples from the past that you have stored in your head to use as evidence at some stage.

This technique is called 'broken record'. Its basic principles are:

1. State what you want and how you feel, if appropriate.
2. Listen to the person's reply, and let them know you have heard and understood them.
3. Repeat your statement or request.

The tyranny of thinness is a form of oppression

I have talked a lot about the tyranny of thinness and oppression. Oppression is one-way mistreatment of one group of individuals within that group by others. In a fat-phobic society, thinner people are in a position to oppress fatter people. This can be anything from an apparently throwaway comment about a person's size, through inappropriate healthcare and lack of positive images of people larger than size 12 in the media, to discrimination in employment. Oppressions lend themselves to interlinking with other oppressions – for example, sizeism and sexism where the Duchess of York is vilified in the press and gossiped about in workplaces because of her size, but the Duke of York isn't.

We are not born oppressors – we learn it as we are growing up. Adults often oppress children to cover their own hurts. For example, a disciplinarian attitude with stringent rules and harsh punishments for transgressions may be rooted in similar treatment that an adult received as a child. As children we get hurt by the people we rely on for nurturing. We learn to misdirect our feelings of hurt, fear and anger on to others – and this opens the door for many other oppressions to take hold.

Oppression is communicated through fear and insecurity and perpetuated through:

- denial
- lack of information
- misinformation
- distortion
- assumptions
- stereotypes
- prejudices

The tyranny of thinness is a form of oppression which affects us all and works like this. Imagine two giant pillars holding up a large bridge (oppression). The pillar on the left is made up of oppressors, and the one on the right is made up of the oppressed (see p 211).

The oppressors are the diet industry, advertising, the fashion industry, the media, the education system, the Health Service and so on. The oppressed are men, women and children of all sizes, but especially large sizes.

To be in one group does not automatically exclude you from the other. You can be both oppressor and oppressed. For example, the publisher of diet books who feels her body is 'slug-like' has assimilated the negative messages about her body that she has received through the tyranny, and at the same time she is churning out more and more body-hating diet books. If you don't like your body and are bad-mouthing Fergie – or any other woman – for her body size and shape, you are both oppressor and oppressed.

Even if all oppressors faced up to the fact that they oppressed people, the tyranny would still exist because the oppressed group will have taken seriously the negative messages about themselves. Given the prevalence of the tyranny of thinness, most of us operate in both groups much of the time.

Healing the effects of the tyranny

Think about the following:

As oppressed

What have I absorbed about myself in the subordinate position?

It is hoped that some of the skills and techniques suggested in this book will contribute towards healing the effects of being oppressed (tyrannized), so that when we are confronted with oppressors their comments (hurts) do not disempower us.

As oppressor

What have I internalised about myself in the dominant position?

As oppressors we need to look at our behaviour to understand and to begin to heal ourselves, so that when a person attacks oppressors (or me) I can hear or receive their criticisms without being or feeling attacked.

Recognizing where we are and the parts we are playing enables us to choose to make a difference, because the tyranny only works when oppressors and oppressed are both prepared to participate. If we dismantle the pillars, the bridge collapses.

Changing society: effective complaints and boycotts

If you feel a product, advertisement, radio or television programme is detrimental to your wellbeing; if it is prejudiced, biased, unreasonable or unfair; if it puts you and/or other women in a bad light or perpetuates or exacerbates the diet mentality; or if you believe it is an outright con – don't just sigh, grunt and put up with it, or moan to everyone except those who need to change. Do something about it!

Organizations and people change their attitudes and opinions for a variety of reasons, but it is usually a combination of the following:

- Through discussion
- When it becomes easier to change than to continue as before
- When it makes good financial sense

Moaning about something and yet doing nothing about it can make us feel worse because we feed into our feelings of powerlessness. We become victims, and adopt a 'poor me' or 'if only' approach. We can bore the pants off people around us, and they switch off when they hear us bleating away.

Complaining effectively, on the other hand, can be very liberating and can actually achieve results. To be effective you have to ensure that your complaint is heard by the appropriate person or organization. There are a number of organizations whose *raison d'être* is to aid you in airing your complaint; the addresses of those described below will be found in Useful Addresses.

Press Complaints Commission

If you have a complaint about an item in a newspaper or magazine, you may find it helpful to write to the Press Complaints Commission. It has a code of practice which states that all members of the press have a duty to maintain the highest professional and ethical standards, and to safeguard the public's right to know.

The Commission recommends you to write first to the editor of the publication in question, because this is the quickest way of obtaining a correction or apology. Allow at least seven days for a reply to be sent.

If the matter is not settled, or if you are dissatisfied with the response, then you should write to the Commission. If possible, identify the particular clause in the code of practice which you believe has been broken and enclose a dated copy of the item about which you are complaining. Only complaints that can be resolved under the code of practice are dealt with. A booklet called *How to Complain* is available from the Commission.

Independent Television Commission

This organization ITC has codes of practice pertaining to advertising, programmes and sponsorship which programme makers and producers and advertising agencies have to comply with. The ITC Programme Code includes guidance on how programmes should avoid offence to good taste and decency, in terms of their content and scheduling. The Code of Advertising Standards and Practice says that television advertising must not be misleading, must not encourage or condone harmful behaviour, and should not cause widespread or exceptional offence.

BBC (British Broadcasting Corporation)

The BBC has several points of contact for viewers and listeners to give comments, queries or criticism relating to programmes or policy. Contact Viewer and Listener Information (see Useful Addresses). If you believe a programme is badly inaccurate, has seriously invaded privacy or is a breach of broadcasting standards, the Programme Complaints Unit (see Useful Addresses) operates independently of programme departments and aims to ensure that all complaints are investigated. If your complaint is upheld, the BBC will find a way of making appropriate acknowledgement or connection, sometimes on air. If you are not happy with the outcome you can get in touch with the Appeals Committee of the Board of Governors, who are appointed to protect public interest and to ensure that the BBC reflects public interests and needs.

Office of Fair Trading

The OFT aims to protect the consumer by encouraging competition among businesses and making sure that trading practices are as fair as possible. The OFT has three main areas of responsibility:

1. Proposing and promoting changes in law and practice where the interests of consumers are being harmed.

2. Taking legal action where possible against businesses that cause problems for consumers.
3. Equipping consumers with information and advice that they need.

The OFT doesn't take up individual cases, which would be dealt with by the Trading Standards Officer in your local authority.

Institute of Trading Standards Administration

This is the professional body representing the views of Trading Standards Officers around the country. It is able to argue the case to government, the ministries, and trade and industry for adopting certain standards to ensure fair trading and protection for honest traders and consumers.

Advertising Standards Authority

The organization which regulates advertisements in non-broadcast media in the UK by supervising the British Code of Advertising Practice.

Who else can you complain to?

You can also write to the people who are representing you – your MP, MEP and local councillors. Contrary to what you may think, most of those who rely on your vote do pay attention when letters come flooding in. (Rumour has it that Members of Parliament measure their post.) You can write to your local councillor at your town hall. If you are not sure who your elected representatives are, your Town Hall Information Department should be able to help you. It should also be able to tell you where to write to your MEP. You can write to your MP at the House of Commons (see Useful Addresses).

As you see, there are plenty of channels through which complaints can be made. Do use them. Let people know when you are not happy or satisfied with things.

Having said that, it is the easiest thing in the world to complain – but unless we tell people how things can be different, they may never learn, so when you give your criticism make sure your complaint is accompanied with a suggestion on how to improve things. For example, 'I am ringing up to complain about . . . (describe the situation) because . . . (the effect). I would like to suggest . . . .'

Positive feedback

If you particularly enjoy a television programme, appreciate a new approach at your local health centre, are pleased with the latest fashion lines in your local department store – tell 'em. Write to the appropriate person – the managing director, the customer service unit – and tell them that you like it. Follow these three simple steps:

- Tell them specifically what you like
- Ask them to continue the good practice
- Thank them

Most of us flourish under praise, so encourage them to flourish the way we want them to!

From little acorns . . .

Never forget that you have power: both personal power and purchasing power. There are several quick and easy ways to get your message across, to let people know you are dissatisfied with their message or their products. One is to write and tell them. Another is to tell your friends and colleagues. And a third is to stop spending your money with any organization that perpetuates the tyranny of thinness and the diet mentality. Such acts are very empowering and really do have effect.

Two of the most successful product boycotts were the South African and the Tuna-Dolphin campaigns. For more than twenty years millions of people, myself included, did not buy South African produce as a way of saying 'no' to apartheid. Sometimes it was a pain in the neck. Sometimes it was the only produce on the greengrocer's stall which meant doing without or going elsewhere in the hope of buying fruit from another country. However, the feeling of empowerment that I got from boycotting made it worthwhile and actually quite easy.

At first some people thought I was mad.

'Oh,' they said, 'it'll never make any difference. What's the point?'

Well, there were several points. Firstly, I was not the only one. Millions of other people were boycotting, too. The ANC have since said they felt a sense of solidarity from people in other countries, knowing we were protesting as best we could against the racist South African regime. Secondly, the boycott and sanctions played a significant part in persuading the South African government that change was necessary – and, in the long run, their best option. Thirdly, I FELT BETTER. I gained a sense of self-respect in the knowledge that I was acknowledging my personal outrage and disapproval of this intolerable regime at the same time as making a contribution towards change for the better. If it can overthrow the tyranny of apartheid, surely we can overthrow the tyranny of thinness.

Open letter to all women

Dear Colleague

I am asking for your help. You may be a Member of Parliament, a teacher, a local councillor, a personnel officer, a social worker, a typist, an administrator, a factory worker, a counsellor, a shop assistant, a trade union member or officer, a doctor, a nurse, an osteopath, a homeopath, a psychotherapist, a sister, a cousin, an aunt, a mother, a grandmother, a writer, a TV personality, a producer, an editor, a company director, a vicar – whatever your role, you are in a unique position of power to do something to destroy the diet mentality. Your contribution could be large or small, depending on your position. It doesn't matter – all contributions are welcome.

If you are a teacher, organize a project in your school around the issues of dieting and positive self-image. Mothers, you can help your daughters (and sons) to develop a positive self-image and protect them from the diet mentality. Perhaps you are a doctor: make sure your patients know about the perils and futility of dieting, and provide information about a healthy lifestyle that is motivating and supportive. If you are involved in politics, support MP Alice Mahon's efforts to regulate the diet industry and her Early Day Motions in support of International No Diet Day. At local level, encourage your authority to be involved via education, health and leisure services, exhibitions in libraries and so on. Company directors, personnel officers, writers, TV personalities, producers: use your positions to influence your staff, your readers, your viewers and the general public. Stop the plethora of dieting items on your shows.

We can release ourselves – from the tyranny of thinness and her chum fat phobia, and so begin to learn a different and better way of relating to ourselves and other women. We have the power to do this, and really it is very easy. Think – what can I do today to help? Do something to make yourself feel better, and something to improve things for others.

Please use your power – for yourself and for the benefit of all women. Together we can do it – and we deserve it!

Whatever you do may seem insignificant, but it is most important that you do it.

Gandhi

9

We Deserve Better – and We Are Going to Have Better!

You are entering a No Dieting area . . .

The degree to which the tyranny of thinness has affected and influenced society is reflected in the number and diversity of anti-diet supporters. As the evidence against dieting mounts, so the anti-diet movement has gained momentum over the last few years. Now thousands of people around the world are united in the common aim of working towards self-acceptance and genuine good health.

I see parallels with the anti-smoking movement. Twenty-five or thirty years ago smoking was socially acceptable. It was portrayed as sophisticated and sexy. Celebrities would smoke as they were interviewed on television, and in films the signal for satisfactory sex was a couple lighting up at the end of the love scene. It was such an ordinary everyday habit that children grew up expecting to smoke, and just as girls now start dieting to demonstrate their advancement into womanhood, we took to fags to show we were now grown up.

Nobody asked if it was OK to smoke when we visited each other's homes. Meetings and workplaces were thick with smoke, as were shops and waiting rooms. If a person protested it was they who seemed odd, not the smokers. In those days people would say that a cigarette after eating helped them digest their food. They were not joking, and nobody laughed.

A lot has changed in the intervening years. Not everyone has stopped smoking, of course, but it is no longer socially acceptable. Many organizations have a no-smoking policy in the workplace and sponsor non-smoking workshops for their employees, and the country now has an annual No Smoking Day to raise awareness and to help more people stop smoking. People do now ask if it's OK to light up, and even smokers will accept that there is a health hazard to themselves and to those around them.

As the facts about dieting become better known and the anti-diet movement gains strength, public opinion will change. Dieting will not be regarded as normal behaviour. Weight loss will not be recommended as the panacea for good health. Consenting adults will diet if they want to, but fewer people *will* want to – just those hanging on to old habits.

The anti-diet movement

The movement is made up of a wide range of individuals and organizations:

- *Women* who are spurning the tyranny of thinness.
- *Politicians* who are concerned about people's health and well-being and are demanding better consumer rights pertaining to diet products.
- *Academics and researchers* who repudiate the claims of weight loss companies and the efficacy of many of their products and methods.
- *Eating disorder specialists* who link dieting to severe eating disorders such as anorexia and bulimia
- *Parents and teachers* who are concerned about young children and teenagers dieting.
- *Consumer organizations* who want greater consumer rights where weight loss products are concerned.
- *Trading Standards and Fair Trading officials* who are concerned about the false claims made by weight loss organizations.
- *Size activists* who are unhappy and angry at the oppression that a diet culture causes them.
- *Food campaigners and researchers* who are dissatisfied at the content of diet foods and products.
- *Governments* who want to take an active lead against dieting and to advocate a healthy, active lifestyle.

As you would expect, the movement is not spread evenly across the globe, and its strength in any particular country does not necessarily reflect the size of the diet industry there. In America, for example, the anti-diet movement is large and strong – but so is the diet industry.

The movement has progressed remarkably quickly and we have made some significant achievements, sometimes moving two steps forward and one step back, but advancing none the less. As we make progress or fill a gap in one area, so we spot another need somewhere else. Britain's Health Service is a good example.

Where we are in Britain

Doctors now know the damage that yo-yo dieting can cause – it is at last recognized, along with anorexia and bulimia, as an eating disorder – and appreciate that many of their patients have tried their damnedest to diet and lose weight but without long-term success. Many doctors are setting up their own clinics within surgeries to support patients. Admittedly some clinics are still offering diet sheets and GPs are still sending patients to slimming organizations, but an increasing number are not. What's more, many doctors now refer patients to Diet Breakers, and some doctors are themselves members and subscribe to our magazine, *Db*.

However, at the same time as increasing numbers of doctors are questioning the validity of putting patients on diets, some of their colleagues in the Health Service, backed up by Health Secretary Virginia Bottomley, are refusing health treatment to fat people. Other officials are drawing up 'healthy eating guidelines' which, according to Lyndel Costain, spokeswoman for the British Dietetic Association, are no inducement to change the unhealthy dietary habits of a lifetime.

Government pressures

Under the health promotion scheme introduced by the British government in spring 1994, doctors are encouraged to advise patients on their lifestyles. On the surface this sounds a good thing, but the implication is that those who fail to conform to healthy lifestyle standards may be refused NHS care for their 'self-inflicted' diseases, and there have been several cases reported in the press of doctors refusing to treat fat people and smokers. Paula wrote to us, 'I weigh 17½ stone – when I first started dieting, many years ago, I only weighed 14 stone! Now my doctor is refusing to treat me until I lose weight. Yes, it's true – and I am not the only ample lassie he has said this to.'

Few doubt that doctors and healthcare professionals are concerned about the health of the British people. But the government's enthusiasm for the concept of healthier lifestyles has as much to do with money as with conviction.

Many of the steps that the government is urging can be taken at local GP level rather than at the more expensive hospital and consultancy stage. GPs have been issued with the *Better Living, Better Life* handbook, which spells out the government's desired lifestyle changes. And since 1993 National Health contracts have been offering higher payments to GPs prepared to tackle patients' unhealthy lifestyles. Virginia Bottomley is convinced that reducing the level of obesity in adults is one way of lowering the incidence of heart disease and stroke. Consequently, doctors will be urging people to lose weight whether they want to or not. *Better Living, Better Life* accepts that it is not feasible for doctors constantly to monitor the progress of all overweight patients and suggests that practice nurses, self-help groups and commercial organizations like Weight Watchers can help. There are no recommendations on how the health of dieters can be monitored, and the perils of yo-yo dieting are not mentioned.

Those targeted are the most overweight (those with a BMI of 30+), those with perceived risk factors for heart disease and stroke, and those with medical conditions thought to be made worse by being overweight. In *Better Living, Better Life*, under Section 5, 'Healthy Eating and Sensible Drinking for CHD [coronary heart disease] and Stroke Prevention', step 6 on page 21 advises doctors to urge people in the targeted categories to go on a diet of 800–1599 kCal (calories) a day. But if an individual's weight loss should 'plateau' on this semi-starvation regime, asserts the final paragraph of step 6, additional calorie restriction may then be required. Is this medicine – or murder?

The dieting truths that the British government ignores

So government experts are recommending diets of as few as 800 calories a day. But some nutritionists believe that any diet of normal foodstuffs (rather than special formula diets) of less than 1200 kCal a day is unlikely to provide all the nutrients that the body needs, and research by Ancel Keyes showed alarming physical and mental effects of semi-starvation on a group of willing, young, healthy volunteers who were limited to 1570 kCal a day. The authorities in other countries, too, are backing this view. US State of Michigan guidelines, for instance, recommend hospital in-patient treatment for those going on a diet of 800 kCal a day or less. In 1989 the Canadian Task Force on the Treatment of Obesity issued the following warnings:

> *Nutritionally deficient programs.* It must be assumed that diets of less than 1200 calories per day based on regular foods will not provide sufficient vitamins, minerals and nutrients to meet an individual's requirements. Nonetheless, these diets are being used in some treatment programs, without the necessary supervision of physicians and dietitians.
> *Diets less than 900 calories.* Very low calorie diets should be provided only under medical supervision by a doctor specially trained to treat obesity, working with an interdisciplinary team of health professionals. This may not always be the case at present.

The British government appears to be unaware of the growing realization by some American experts that a fat person who has lost weight is not the same as a person who has always been that (lower) weight. Reports indicate that those who have slimmed may be at more risk from heart disease than fat people who have never dieted.

Meanwhile, Dr Anne Walker and Professor Isle of Glasgow University have made discoveries which contradict the government gospel – but their results received less attention than they deserved. Within weeks of the government launching its scheme Walker and Isle called a press conference to publicize their findings:

- that obesity was not independently correlated with coronary heart disease mortality in a fifteen-year follow-up study
- that the highest level of blood cholesterol in women carried less risk than the lowest level in men
- and that a low fat, cholesterol-lowering diet as recommended for men may not be appropriate for women

Professor John Garrow is the UK's leading expert on 'obesity'; he has been working in the field for almost thirty years. By his own admission the success rate for treating obesity (making obese people permanently thin) is very disappointing. If it doesn't work for John Garrow, I wonder why Virginia Bottomley thinks GPs will be more successful.

A sceptic could be forgiven for thinking that the government's health scheme had more to do with weeding out 'undeserving' patients in an under-funded Health Service. After all, which group is less politically organized than fat people? So who is less 'deserving'?

Nevertheless, despite the official line, there are some torch-bearers out there among the movers and shakers in Britain. For a number of years individuals from the ranks of eating disorder specialists, other health professionals, researchers and politicians have been talking and working actively against dieting, aware of the links between it and more serious eating disorders. Certain people from these professions have supported Diet Breakers consistently since we started. We still need to forge links with 'obesity experts' in Britain who support a non-diet approach (See page 62 for a medical definition of obesity). There must be some out there; disappointingly, we haven't found them yet.

Why I started Diet Breakers

In the autumn of 1991 I started running workshops for women which I called Do You Really Need to Diet? They sprang from the Developing Women's Management Potential courses that I run. During one women's management course we broke for coffee and the usual chit-chat started when the biscuits came round. You know the kind of thing . . . 'Oh, I'll have just one', 'I shouldn't really', 'Oh, all right then'. Of course, like all of us, I'd heard it all hundreds of times before. But this particular day I became irritated. I listened to the ensuing conversation about the biscuits and the diets, and when we returned from the break I asked the group, 'What do you think would happen if you spent as much time and energy on your careers (which was why we were together) as you do on diets?'

It was as if I had struck a match. Everyone wanted to discuss it and everyone had something to say. Suddenly it dawned on me that there was a real problem, with powerful influences underpinning it. Several people suggested I run some workshops based on this issue; they were immediately over-subscribed, with long waiting lists.

Then I saw a television programme in which three women were having their stomachs stapled in an effort to become thin. None of them received any counselling before undergoing this major surgery. One of the women had split her staples, regained the weight and undergone the operation again – three times. I found this programme unbelievably distressing: the physical and emotional pain of these women and the depth of their self-loathing was more than I could bear. I started crying, and went on all night. It was not until the morning that it dawned on me: I was crying for myself too. I had experienced that deep self-loathing.

About a month later I read a newspaper report about a teenager who had hanged herself. She was size 14. Something had to be done, and in the absence of anybody else taking a lead, I decided it would be me. I realized we needed to launch a national campaign drawing attention to the perils and futility of dieting.

Starting to spread the message

In May 1992 I introduced the first No Diet Day. It was originally intended to be National No Diet Day; then, a week before the event, International Clear Your Desk Day was declared as a promotional stunt. Although the event didn't encourage me to clear my desk, it did inspire me to think of No Diet Day as an international event!

I knew the event wouldn't take off overnight. So the first International No Diet Day was a small affair to be celebrated by a dozen of us with a picnic in Hyde Park. It reminded me of my Sunday School outings as a child. There was a buzz of excitement and adventure in the air. We were all dressed up in our best summer outfits and eagerly anticipated tucking into our picnic spread, which looked and tasted wonderful. We had all brought food and drink to share – a glorious array of cheeses and crusty breads, pâtés, smoked salmon, salads, soups, pies, chicken, fruit, cakes, trifle, fruit juice, beer, wine and champagne. The youngest woman in our party was twenty-one, the oldest seventy-six, and we all wore stickers saying: DITCH THAT DIET. The media turned up in force and jostled to interview us and take photographs.

Unfortunately the English weather had its own agenda that day. Pavarotti was not the only person rained out of Hyde Park in the summer of 1992. But the weather didn't quell our enthusiasm and we ended up having the picnic in my living room, with the media sheltering under umbrellas queuing to come in.

There was a mixture of inquisitiveness, amusement, bewilderment and contempt. Some journalists genuinely wanted to find out more about us, others had been sent along by their papers to look for a 'light-hearted' story, while yet others were there to be rude and poke fun. Whatever their angle, they all wanted to know the same thing: what we anti-diet people actually looked like, what exactly we believed in if we didn't believe in diets, and, even more important, what did we eat? The journalists' questions demonstrated how we have all been seduced by the diet mentality. Many of their questions could have been thought up by the industry itself: 'Are you going to be "stuffing yourselves" with chip butties, doughnuts and cream cakes?', 'What's wrong – don't you like lettuce and cottage cheese?', 'Aren't you afraid of getting fat?', 'Do you think all doctors have got it wrong?', 'But obesity can't be healthy for you!', and so on. We made the national and local radio, press and television, and thousands of women wrote in to Diet Breakers wanting to know more.

Friends – and foes – in high places

By the time the second International No Diet Day came around, in 1993, we had achieved far more than we could have imagined. Diet Breakers had made a half-hour television programme as part of BBC's *Open Door* series, we had given hundreds of media interviews, taken part in debates at universities and given

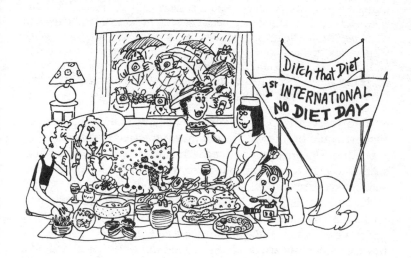

presentations to a wide range of organizations. We had also gained the support of a very important ally: Alice Mahon, Member of Parliament for Halifax.

Alice has been untiring in supporting and championing the aims and work of Diet Breakers. In 1993 and again in 1994 she presented to the House of Commons this Early Day Motion in support of International No Diet Day:

That this House supports International No Diet Day on 5th May, the purpose of which is to draw attention to the perils and futility of dieting, except for medical reasons such as stomach ulcers and diabetes, and to promote a healthier way of living; notes that dieting undermines people's emotional and physical wellbeing and is often the first step towards more serious eating disorders; condemns the pressure on women, girls and young men to be unhealthily thin; is concerned that dieting has reached epidemic levels; notes that 90 per cent of women will diet at some time in their lives, and at any given time 50 per cent of women are dieting, including girls as young as eight years and women as old as 75 years; regrets that Western women and girls are starving through dieting when in other parts of the world so many people are dying through starvation; believes that the tyranny of thinness encourages women to be valued on their looks alone and encourages the oppression of fat people as well as causing misinformation on healthy living and eating; realizes that, whilst obesity may cause health risks to some people, the solution is not a simple one of losing weight because 96 per cent of diets do not work, and dieting causes other problems including low self-esteem, mood swings, depression, gall stones, lack of concentration, constipation and headaches; and therefore supports International No Diet Day for a better way of living.

Seventy-three Members of Parliament added their signature in support of the EDM in 1993, and they supported it again in 1994.

In 1993 we organized a lunch and afternoon forum on that special day. It was led by Sue Dibb from the Food Commission, who spoke about her research into diet products, and Dr Bridget Dolan from St George's Medical School and the European Council on Eating Disorders. In the intervening year we had forged links with campaigners in the USA, Canada and elsewhere, and the day was celebrated in various places around the world. We adopted a pale blue ribbon as our symbol of solidarity for the day.

By the time we came to celebrate the third anniversary, in 1994, International No Diet Day was observed in most major cities of the USA, all the Canadian provinces, New Zealand, Australia, Moscow, Ireland and Europe. In addition, nearly forty events were held throughout Britain which celebrated the day in a variety of ways: a lone woman worker left a box of chocolates by the photocopier with an open invitation for all to help themselves and enjoy the day, a number of schools organized projects, a sumptuous lunch for fifty women in Wiltshire raised money for a bereavement charity, and students in Newcastle wrapped themselves in tape measures and held a debate.

In central London, Diet Breakers and Alice Mahon held a press conference at the House of Commons where we were supported by Professor Tom Sanders of Kings College, co-author of the excellent book *You Don't Have to Diet*, and again by Bridget Dolan. Later there was a lobby of Parliament, and the day was nicely rounded off with a large rally in the evening. The evening consisted of a mix of music, entertainment and speeches, and was attended by women of all sizes, ages and cultural backgrounds.

The day before No Diet Day, MP Tony Banks introduced a Ten Minute Rule Bill calling for an end to job discrimination on the

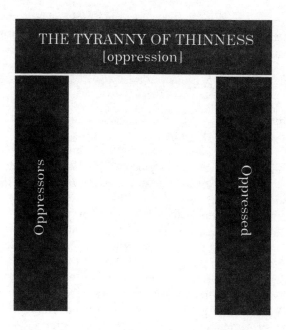

THE TYRANNY OF THINNESS
[oppression]

Oppressors

Oppressed

basis of size, which received much publicity. Tony cited a number of examples where he said prejudice had taken place, including his own researcher trying to get a job with Virgin Airlines. Although the timing of his Bill in relation to No Diet Day was purely coincidental, we were all able to exploit the media opportunities to demonstrate the links between the pressure to diet and size oppression.

A month later Alice Mahon introduced a Ten Minute Rule Bill to Regulate the Diet Industry. The aims of the Bill were based on legislation that New York City has introduced:

- All weight loss centres prominently to display a health warning that rapid weight loss is dangerous to health.
- All weight loss companies to provide all consumers with a card which clearly outlines the benefits and the risks of weight loss.
- All weight loss companies to disclose additional charges that the consumer may incur for the purchase of products, laboratory tests etc.
- All diet and weight loss pills and potions to be brought under the Medicines Act.

- All products, including books, tapes and videos, to state clearly that permanent weight loss is unlikely and cannot be guaranteed.
- Weight loss providers to tell consumers what the actual or estimated duration of the recommended programme will be.

Unfortunately the government was against the Bill. Michael Fabricant, Conservative MP for Mid-Staffordshire opposed it under the misguided conviction that 'The ten thousand slimming club leaders in Britain perform a valuable service to the community and make a positive contribution to the nation's health because 50 per cent of adults in the country are overweight and diet products are not only safe, but are often extremely succcessful.'

Unfortunately he did not explain how he measured success or where his figures had come from. When Rosemary Conley and I appeared together on the *Kilroy* TV show she claimed that 50 per cent of the nation are overweight, and this is where the confusion comes in with the interchangeability of the words 'overweight' and 'obese'. In terms of health risk, the present government states in its health policy document, *The Health of the Nation*, its target of reducing obesity from the current level of 13–16 per cent to less than 6 per cent. Tom Sanders and Peter Bazalgette say that people with a BMI of 25–30 are in the low risk groups, but according to many in the diet industry a BMI of 25 constitutes being overweight. It is shocking to think that the evidence is being ignored.

Confusing the facts has led to thousands of women in low health risk groups, myself included, being wrongly advised that they should lose weight for health reasons. And, given how the efficacy of weight loss programmes is so limited, and the associated health risks of such programmes so great, I believe it is even more shocking that the government appears to promote them to those people who *may* be at risk.

The dangers for children

Recent research shows that many children are snacking rather than having proper meals, they are eating too much sugar and fat, and they are not getting enough fruit and vegetables. According to B.E. Livingstone in *CHO International Dialogue* (Vol. II, issue

2, 1991), increased consumption of convenience and snack foods now amounts to one-third of a child's energy intake. Some children, however, have gone to the other extreme: taking the nutritional advice at face value, they have cut out fat altogether and developed the unhelpful notion of 'good' and 'bad' food. Children, affected by the cultural wisdom of the slim and body-beautiful, are now dieting as young as six and seven. Since 1994 was the Year of the Family, we used the opportunity to launch our Diet Breakers' Health and Diet Roadshow for Children. We want to help prevent children falling prey to the diet trap and developing negative body images. It is our modest attempt to fight back against the diet industry's influence on children.

In the two years since the inception of Diet Breakers I have recruited a team of country-wide facilitators to run our ten-week programme called You Count, Calories Don't. It is based on Canadian dietician Linda Omichinski's book of the same name. Diet Breakers' facilitators are committed to fighting the tyranny of thinness, and as part of our campaigning work we talk and work with parents and teachers' groups, women's organizations and children, providing information, motivation and support for them to develop projects with the children in their care.

Size matters

Another of our campaigns is for standard British clothing sizes. Shopping for clothes can be a nightmare for women trapped in the diet mentality. Having absorbed the message that certain dress sizes are more desirable than others, having to buy a dress or skirt in a larger size is horrendous. Indeed, many women decide not to buy the garment, preferring to 'wait until they've lost weight'.

The paradox is that, whilst women are attempting to mould their bodies to fit certain sizes, many garments are not accurately labelled. Manufacturers can, and do, 'massage' their sizes so much that we have grown quite used to it. How many times have you heard comments along the lines '. . . This manufacturer's clothes come up big' or 'I always take a size smaller in . . .'? We discovered that manufacturers can label their skirts and dresses as any size they like because, unlike with shoes, gloves and hats, there is no standard sizing. So Diet Breakers and Alice Mahon launched a campaign calling for Standard British Dress Sizing.

The size range for women's clothing in Britain was set more than forty years ago. Women aged sixteen to sixty were measured in the early 1950s. Their average sizes, based on measurements taken from three points on the body, became the familiar 12, 14, 16, 18, 20, 22, 24, 26 etc. sizing.

At the time of the original survey women had been through World War II, and some had gone through World War I as well. During the forties and into the fifties there was rationing in Britain. Women's lifestyles then were very different from those of today's women. We now eat different food, we eat out more, we diet more, we walk less, we have modern labour-saving conveniences, and we work outside the home more than we did in the fifties (if not during the war).

Today's women are better nourished and enjoy better health care. Some have been made bigger by continued dieting. We tend to have bigger and lower breasts, thicker waists, larger upper hips, a more rounded tummy, fatter upper arms and a bigger ribcage. The traditional hourglass figure – which was, after all, only imposed unnaturally on women's bodies by the late unlamented corset – has been replaced by a rounder body. Yet the majority of clothing manufacturers still base their patterns on the shapes and measurements taken all those years ago.

When Alice Mahon asked the President of the Board of Trade, Michael Heseltine, why there are no standard British dress sizes, he replied: '. . . the Government's view is that the development, promotion and use of Standards is best undertaken by the industry itself, with the support of the British Standard Institution, in the light of consumer requirements in the market, on a voluntary basis'.

Considering the millions of women who are attempting to change their body shape – through dieting and cosmetic surgery – to fit into outdated dress sizes, not to mention the waste of time nipping in and out of the changing room trying to fathom what size we take in any particular store, we believe it is time to label clothes accurately.

The DB Awards

Inspired by political campaigns and magazines in America, if not by the Oscars, Tonys and BAFTAs, Diet Breakers' magazine, *Db*, introduced the annual *Db* Awards. The purpose is to thank and reward people and organizations working to end the tyranny of thinness and who have made an outstanding positive contribution to the anti-diet movement. The categories for the award are:

- Political
- International
- Positive Image
- Book of the Year
- *Db*'s Special Award – a person or organization that deserves special merit
- The *Db* Raspberry – the person or organization who deserves a raspberry for their pro-dieting or anti-self-acceptance stance

Advertising

At the end of 1994 Diet Breakers introduced another on-going campaign, Boycott Anorexic Marketing, which has a counterpart in America. From the responses to our questionnaire we know that advertising has a lot to answer for in terms of women's body dissatisfaction, low self-esteem and dieting habits.

We urge consumers to avoid products that are promoted by unhealthily thin, childlike or vulnerable models and to think twice about buying toys and dolls that give children the message that long and thin equals beautiful, or muscular and macho equals manliness. We are delighted that the Independent Television Commission has proposed scheduling restrictions on slimming products, treatments and establishments being shown immediately adjacent to children's programmes and those likely to appeal to under eighteen-year-old audiences.

Slimming products may also not now be aimed at the clinically obese, since large-scale weight loss should be conducted under close medical supervision and testimonials of weight loss products must not be from people who are, or appear to be, underweight. Regrettably, the ruling does not apply to advertisements for calorie-reduced foods and drinks that don't emphasize slimming or weight control.

The code of practice supervised by the Advertising Standards Authority (see page 197) states that the only way for a person to lose weight is by taking in less energy (calories) than the body is using. So claims which suggest that weight loss can be achieved wholly by any other means contravene the code.

In January 1994 the Authority carried out a one-month spot check survey of all advertisements containing claims for slimming, weight or inch loss and figure control, with the aim of identifying exaggerated or unrealistic claims for these products. The sample covered national daily and Sunday newspapers, women's magazines and the six largest regional newspapers.

The ASA found a total of 124 adverts, including repeat appearances. Analysing the sample showed 31 different ads, 11 of which caused no problem under the code. Of the remaining 20 advertisements, 6 were already the subject of complaint, monitoring or copy advice action and 14 contained potential breaches of the code. The findings represent a problem level of 64.5 per cent, compared to similar spot check surveys relating to car and alcohol advertising which showed problem levels of 10.6 per cent and 3.8 per cent, respectively.

The primary problem revealed was a certain type of advertising that persistently included claims such as: 'Overnight Miracle Slim' and 'No Dieting, No Exercise!' Such advertisers usually resist complying with the code or substantiating their claims by telling the ASA that the advertisement will not appear again. Lamentably, other equally objectionable ads often take their place. So the ASA has to keep constant vigil on the same operators.

Another area of concern for the ASA is advertisements for cosmetic surgery which imply that the effects are permanent and the means of achieving them are simple. The patient is not guaranteed that she will not regain weight; and liposculpture and liposuction involve invasive surgery that carries the associated risks common to all surgery. So claims such as 'Permanent fat removal' and 'A minor outpatient procedure' are not acceptable.

Finally, contrary to the code, some advertisements claim that actual inch/weight loss is achievable through using garments such as 'thinning belts', 'body wraps' or exercise equipment.

Although ASA is keeping an on-going watch on all such misleading advertising, in the long run it may be that self-regulation in the form of a code of practice is not sufficient and that legislation may be needed.

Organizations, magazines, journals and films

For addresses of organizations, or details of where resources may be obtained, see Useful Addresses on page 237.

Britain

Db

You can become a member of Diet Breakers by subscribing to our magazine, *Db*, which is published four times a year. It contains interesting articles, news up dates on dieting and related health and food issues as well as gossip and fun. Membership keeps supporters in touch and helps to fund our campaign work. Db members are given priority at Diet Breakers' events such as the No Diet Day celebrations.

You Count, Calories Don't

In response to so many Diet Breakers' supporters asking for help to stop dieting, we have collaborated with leading Canadian dietitian Linda Omichinski to bring this programme to the UK. It enables you to:

- Identify the difference between emotional and physical hunger and meet your different needs
- Develop a healthy, natural and enjoyable relationship with food
- Incorporate exercise into your life in a non-obsessive way
- Work to achievable and sustainable life-style objectives, not related to weight loss
- Feel good about yourself and your body

For more information about Linda's work, see page 220.

For more information about all Diet Breakers' work, and to find out where your nearest facilitator is, send an A5 stamped addressed envelope to the address given on page 239.

Eating Disorders Association

The largest registered charity offering help and understanding for anorexia and bulimia in Britain. The EDA provides telephone helplines, a bi-monthly members' newsletter, *Signpost*, and self-help groups around the country.

Synergetic workouts

An organization headed by fitness expert and model Astrid Longhurst and her partner Loz McCarthy. Astrid has her own famous yo-yo diet story. Years ago she was 'The Slimcea Girl', and an advertising campaign was built around her successful diet based on Slimcea bread. Fast forward to today, and Astrid is a super-fit size 18–20. Loz is a smaller woman, and together they cut a magnificently positive image of fit at any size. They offer Mind and Body Fitness Programmes for people of all sizes in and around London and the South-East. Astrid is also the fitness expert in *YES*! magazine (see below).

Pretty Big

A quarterly style and fashion magazine for large women, available by subscription.

Fat Women's Group

Monthly support group meetings with a quarterly newsletter, *Fat News*, available by subscription.

YES!

A bi-monthly magazine, available from newsagents, that takes a positive approach to size 16+. It is glossy and very professional and manages to combine all the usual women's magazine items such as fashion, lifestyle, make-overs etc. with more serious articles and contributions from highly regarded writers such as Shelley Bovey and Sherry Ashworth. There are regular items on self-esteem and size acceptance, and the magazine has a clear non-diet approach. Diet Breakers has its own regular page. *YES*! came out strongly against Virginia Bottomley's health care policy which gives doctors the right to refuse fat people medical treatment. You don't have to be size 16+ to read and enjoy *YES*!

The food magazine and the Food Commission

The Food Commission is an independent consumer watchdog on food. It provides independently researched information on the food we eat, to ensure good-quality food for all. The Commission has undertaken a number of research projects on diet products, some of which are mentioned in this book. All of them have been critical of diet food products in some respect. *The Food Magazine* is published quarterly by this organization.

Fat Chance: The Big Prejudice

Produced by the National Film Board of Canada, this film helps keep the message of health at any size in the minds of the public. It is the funny and sensitive story of Rick Zakowich, who started on a diet to lose half his body weight and found all of himself along the way. It can be obtained by mail order in the UK from Alternative View (See Useful Addresses).

Canada

As countries go, the anti-diet movement is well advanced here because it is assisted by a number of government initiatives including a public awareness campaign on radio and television and in newspapers since 1991 and a national anti-diet health scheme which is described below.

Vitality

An innovative, nationwide programme run by Health and Welfare Canada, which grew out of their strategy to promote healthy weight. It recommends focussing on health-enhancing attitudes and behaviour to achieve and maintain a healthy weight, rather than focussing on weight itself, and avoiding activities that exacerbate current social preoccupations with weight and body size.

Vitality is an integrated approach that promotes healthy enjoyable eating, active living, and positive self- and body image. It is designed to encourage individuals to make healthy choices and to create an environment that makes healthy choices easy choices. Its aims are very similar to those of Diet Breakers:

1. *Feeling good.* Being positive about yourself and your body. Accepting that healthy bodies come in all shapes and sizes. You have some control over your life.
2. *Eating well.* Enjoyable and healthy eating. Choosing a variety of foods to meet your nutritional needs and to satisfy personal, social, cultural and economic needs. Moderation in fat, salt and alcohol.
3. *Being active.* Valuing physical activity as an integral and enjoyable part of everyday life.

Efforts are made to forge links between health care professionals, employers, media, fashion, fitness specialists and food industries to encourage support for the programme.

The Vitality programme currently targets adults between the ages of twenty-five and forty-one, recognizing that this age group has a major influence on both young families and social values. It also has a lot of body image and weight problems, and people in this age range are considered to be at increased risk of cancer, diabetes and heart disease.

Vitality intends to target children, as well.

HUGS

A pioneer and leader in the anti-diet movement on an international level is Canadian dietitian and Co-ordinator for International No Diet Day, Linda Omichinski. Linda recognized that diets didn't work for her patients and, through her desire to be part of the solution, not the problem, she set up HUGS. It offers two new life-changing goals to replace weight loss, which is the sole focus of diets and weight loss programmes:

1. Self-acceptance of body and shape.
2. Increased energy and wellbeing by learning how to develop the eating patterns that will produce these results.

The effect of these two goals is lifelong better health. HUGS runs a ten-week, self-esteem-based programme based on the philosophy of *You Count, Calories Don't* – the title of Linda's book. The programme enables participants to develop an alternative perspective to the 'diet mentality' and promotes an independent, non-dieting lifestyle characterized by self-acceptance and self-nourishment.

HUGS' approach on health is to forget the scales, calorie counting and fat gram levels. Learn how to tune into your body for the signals that mean 'enough' and 'more'. Discover individual patterns for food and activity levels that keep you energized. Find the strength to accept yourself as you are, and get on with life.

Support materials are provided for use during and after the programme to reinforce the concepts and help participants take in the ideas. They consist of Linda's book, a set of affirmation tapes to instill positive language, and a fitness video that emphasizes active living and feeling comfortable with body movement.

The HUGS programme is available in Canada, the United States and New Zealand, and from Diet Breakers in the UK.

The film *Fat Chance* (see page 219) is available from the National Film Board of Canada (see Useful Addresses).

Norway

In Norway the government has listened to women's groups and health campaigners, studied the evidence and accepted that there are links between the tyranny of thinness, poor body image, dieting and eating disorders.

The government has recognized that essential promotional and preventive measures require united efforts from all sectors of the health and education departments. They have introduced an ambitious and comprehensive scheme for secondary schools and colleges involving the Board of Health and the Ministry of Education and Research.

The primary goals of the project are to promote good health in the general public as well as prevent and treat illness. The education policy in Norway makes schools responsible for caring for and developing the whole person. They therefore need to play a significant role in preventive health work including counteracting superficial and harmful mass media messages.

The Norwegians understand the pivotal role that culture plays in body image, self-acceptance, dieting and eating disorders, and accept that talking about and dealing with eating disorders in isolation is useless. The scheme recognizes that human beings are affected by their environment, and that schools are a part of that environment. And, just as people with eating disorders have to take responsibility for their recovery, so society has to take responsibility to recover by being aware of what is going on and then working and behaving in accordance with that knowledge.

Apart from producing and sending out materials, teachers, school nurses and others are trained and supported in the prevention of eating disorders, in what to do if symptoms are discovered, and in how to deal with the person concerned.

In a follow-up project in Buskerud County, managed by Runi Borresen Gresho, the need was identified for still further professional training and improved coordination between different professionals and institutions. This work has now been established in Buskerud, with the goal of nationwide implementation at a later date (see National Education Office under Useful Addresses).

IKS (Association for Women with Eating Disorders)

IKS is a nationwide self-help organization with several local units and a substantial number of members. Their aims are:

1. To spread information about eating disorders, so that they are treated seriously.
2. To support and aid women with eating disorders, as well as their family and friends.
3. To persuade the public health service to establish adequate and wide-ranging treatment facilities.

IKS has a members' journal, *Kvinnekraft* (*Women's Power*), which offers information, workshops, courses and lectures. There is also a telephone helpline and advice on public health and legal rights.

Norwegian Anorexia/Bulimia Association

Provides support and information to sufferers, relatives, friends and the media. It also organizes local support groups, meetings, seminars and workshops.

USA

At about the same time as I was launching Diet Breakers in Britain, I read about women out on the streets in America protesting that diets don't work and smashing scales, brandishing a slogan: 'Scales are for Fish'. They were fortunate to have their claims supported by the National Institute of Health (NIH).

However, the NIH wasn't always that supportive, as Miriam Berg, President of the Council on Size and Weight Discrimination, explained to me:

The NIH is part of the Federal Government which oversees funding for scientific research on health issues. There are many institutes within the NIH, such as the National Heart, Blood and Lung which, as part of its brief, has jurisdiction over obesity research. The NIH hold consensus panels or technology assessment panels and publish pronouncements which have an important effect on the press, on scientists, and on public opinion.

In 1985 they assembled a group of 'hardline' experts and pronounced obesity a 'killer disease'. Then they studied weight-loss surgery. Unfortunately the only doctors who testified were surgeons themselves, and their follow-up on patients was negligible. The result was a declaration that weight loss surgery was 'safe and effective'.

Activists were fired into response. They got involved with the conference, and provided extensive written testimony. Some supporters were invited to speak at the public input section of the next conference, and in 1991 the NIH investigated dieting and found it to be ineffective.

Even more important, the NIH included a statement opposing size discrimination in the preamble to the panel report. This NIH report has been a great help in convincing the American public that diets don't work.

Since 1991, the American Federal Trade Commission (FTC) has been investigating the claims made by medically supervised and commercial diet programmes in their campaign against deceptive advertising. In December 1993 the FTC gave final approval to consent agreements with Physicians Weight Loss Centres of America, Inc., Diet Center, Inc and Nutri/System, Inc. The three separate agreements settle charges that these marketers of commercial diet programmes made unsubstantiated weight-loss and weight-loss maintenance claims, used consumer testimonials without substantiation that they represented the typical experience of dieters on programmes, and engaged in other false or deceptive advertising practices. The Commission's action makes the consent order provisions binding on the respondents. All three companies are prohibited from misrepresenting the performance or safety of any weight-loss programme they offer in the future and are required to have scientific data to back up future claims they make about weight loss and maintenance. In addition maintenance success claims in most advertisements must be accompanied by various clear and prominent disclosures, for example the statement 'For many dieters, weight loss is temporary' or 'This result is not typical' must be included.

Jenny Craig and Weight Watchers were included in charges that they, like the companies already mentioned, were unable to substantiate claims that their customers typically are successful in reaching their weight loss goals or maintaining them long term. However, Jenny Craig and Weight Watchers are litigating and, at present, the case is awaiting a trial date.

The FTC issues consent agreements for public comment and for settlement purposes only which do not constitute admission of a law violation. When the FTC issues a consent order on a final basis, it carries the force of law with respect to future actions by the respondents. Each violation of such an order may result in a civil penalty of up to $10,000.

According to diet market analyst John Larosa, in the USA the industry has been in recession since 1990. In 1994 the top eleven commercial companies operated 14 per cent fewer centres than in 1991, and in 1991 there were 10 per cent fewer than in 1989. However, the industry is on the road to recovery and expecting to grow 5.3 per cent annually, with revenues of $38.6 billion by 1996.

To counter this trend, there are hundreds of organizations and individuals working in the anti-diet and size acceptance movement in the USA. Many of them have been active in making No Diet Day the international event it has become.

Healthy Weight Journal

A bi-monthly magazine edited by Frances M. Berg that is essential reading for all health professionals and researchers, as well as being interesting and useful for the rest of us. It offers up-to-date news, information and research.

Healthy Weight Journal has also launched a number of campaigns including the Healthy Weight, Healthy Look Contest, whose winners are announced in January each year. The purpose is for members of the American public to send a message to corporate America that they are sick of the advertising industry portraying American women as anorexic, shallow and more absorbed with how they look than with how they feel. Nominations are sought for:

1. Best Business Advertisement
2. Best Fashion Industry Models/Catalogues
3. Best TV Network or Show

Non Diet Workshops

These are run by several organizations, including Diet/Weight Liberation, the Chicago Center for Overcoming Overeating, and GUIDE (Guidance for Image, Dieting, and Eating).

HUGS

Over 30 affiliates across America run the excellent You Count, Calories Don't programme (see under Canada, page 221). Activity video and affirmation tapes also available.

Largely Positive

Under its founder-president, Carol A. Johnson, this organization promotes health, self-esteem and wellbeing among large people. Its activities include a quarterly newsletter, *On a Positive Note*, weekly support groups and periodic workshops. It also provides education on issues of size and weight to professionals such as doctors, therapists, dietitians and fitness personnel.

Body Trust

Under its director, Dayle Hayes, Body Trust runs non-diet workshops and has produced an hour-long video aimed at helping to end body hate, crazy diets and compulsive workouts. It has a three-step approach: feed your body, move your body, love your body.

National Center for Overcoming Overeating

Workshops for over-eaters, based on the book *Overcoming Overeating*, by Jane Hirshman and Carol Munter.

ANRED (Anorexia Nervosa and Related Eating Disorders)

Runs groups for people with eating disorders and those who work with them.

AHELP

A multi-disciplinary organization, under the directorship of Joe McVoy, which is at the leading edge in professional and social education about the inappropriateness and dangers of weight reduction dieting. It holds an annual professional conference, and produces a quarterly newsletter and resource materials.

Largesse

An excellent resource and information clearing house for size diversity empowerment, with a refreshingly clear feminist/libertarian perspective; it maintains a database and archives and offers support materials. Its director is Karen Stimson.

Radiance

A quarterly magazine edited by Alice Ansfield and available on subscription, it contains news and features of interest to women who are 'all sizes of large'. *Radiance* also organize holidays to exciting and different places.

Rump Parliament

A bi-monthly size activist magazine working to change the way society treats fat people. Editor Lee Martindale persuaded Ann Richards, Governor of Texas, to proclaim support for International No Diet Day. Lucky Texas – a diet-free zone! Lee Martindale is also US Co-ordinator of International No Diet Day.

NAAFA (National Association to Advance Fat Acceptance)

Established in 1969, NAAFA campaigns on a national level, holds social events and an annual convention, and produces a newsletter for its members. There are chapters across America and Canada, most of whom organize local events throughout the year and celebrations on No Diet Day.

Council on Size and Weight Discrimination Inc.

An anti-size discrimination group that influences policy and public opinion through education, information and networking. It also provides funding for the International No Diet Day Coalition.

Fat Lip Readers' Theater

Finally, in the American listings, if you're in the San Francisco Bay area keep an eye out for the excellent Fat Lip Readers' Theater. Many of the sketches in their productions have anti-diet themes and are presented with a combination of insight, feelings, political awareness and fun. If they're giving a performance, don't miss it!

Australia

About 300,000 Australians buy weight loss programmes every year from an industry estimated to be worth $500 million annually. In April 1994 Trevor Griffin, the Minister of Consumer Affairs, launched the Voluntary Code of Practice for South Australia's weight control industry, which may serve as a model for the other Australian states.

The code, which is specifically aimed at weight loss centres, fitness centres, health food stores, pharmacists and multi-level marketing organizations and their distributors, addresses significant market problems that cause client disputes or distort fair trading. It was prepared by a consultative committee made up of health professionals, dietitians, counsellors, the Office of Fair Trading and representatives from the weight control industry. The code specifies the following 'Agreed Principles':

- The nutritional value and contents of packaged foods, liquid meal replacement formulae and weight control products are to be disclosed fully on the products.
- Advertisements are to contain a warning that weight change for a person may vary under some circumstances.
- That full health and lifestyle checks, including a screening assessment, will be conducted with clients who want to participate in a weight loss programme.
- That clients suspected of having an eating disorder such as anorexia, bulimia or compulsive eating and those in obvious poor health will not be advised to enter into a weight reduction programme or diet, or be offered dietary food, without a proper referral from a doctor or other appropriate health professional.
- That clients under the age of eighteen will not be encouraged to participate in a weight control programme or to purchase packaged diet foods, liquid meal replacements or weight control products without a letter of referral from a doctor or without the consent of parents or guardians.
- That operators will have access to a range of referral sources.
- Operators are to ensure that consultants don't use harsh or unreasonable or unfair methods of selling weight loss products to clients.
- Operators are to ensure that their consultants don't provide misleading information to prospective clients in an attempt to sell them goods or services.
- All contracts will set out in full and in clear English all contractual terms, including the total costs to be paid.
- Clients will be given a copy of their contract immediately after signing.
- Contracts will be subject to a cooling-off period of three days, starting on and including the day on which the contract was made.
- Contracts will contain, immediately above the space provided for the client's signature, the statement 'THIS CONTRACT IS SUBJECT TO A COOLING-OFF PERIOD OF THREE DAYS', printed in upper case letters in type no smaller than 18 points (which means big!)
- Operators are to have an official refund policy that is made clear to clients at the time of purchasing a weight control programme or product and again on any subsequent enquiries.

- Operators are to have a clear, uniform dispute resolution policy made available to consultants and clients at the point of sale.
- Operators will ensure that consultants are trained adequately to give correct and proper advice to clients.

At present this is a voluntary code, not legislation. Feedback on whether operators are complying with the agreed principles is being monitored.

Australia has its own Why Weight? Body Image and Eating Disorders Awareness Week, celebrated in October. The week offers courses and workshops on self-esteem, health, discrimination, food issues and personal image as well as films, discussion groups and activity events.

Women at Large

Runs anti-diet and self-esteem workshops and publishes a quarterly newsletter, *Life Size*. Under its director, Kathy Sandown, Women at Large aims to raise awareness about fat prejudice and challenge the 'fat stereotype'. Kathy is also Australian co-ordinator of International No Diet Day.

Anorexia and Bulimia Nervosa Foundation of Victoria

Offers a telephone/written information, indirect referral and support service for anyone affected by anorexia or bulimia. Concentrates on the State of Victoria, but is also able to give general information.

New Zealand

There is strong awareness at government level of the need for change and education on the issues of dieting and body image, and a review of mental health policy is under way. Anti-diet activists have been invited to contribute.

The New Zealand Trust for the Prevention of Sub-Clinical Eating Disorders promotes public recognition of the health hazards associated with dieting and the development of an environment where body size and shape diversity is seen as healthy and normal. Set up by women with personal/professional ties with dieting and eating issues, the objective of the Trust is to research and publicize accurate information about the effects of dieting, weight loss and weight management programmes on the physical and mental health of New Zealanders. The Trust advocates regulatory measures that provide protection for diet industry consumers and supports the development of educational programmes, resources and information which promote body acceptance, size-acceptance and self-acceptance.

A number of organizations in New Zealand offer workshops and programmes to help break the diet cycle and promote good health.

Transitions

Offers half-day and one-day workshops and seminars on why diets don't work, and is the New Zealand distributors of the ten-weekly HUGS programme. Director Tania Coombs is also New Zealand Co-ordinator of International No Diet Day.

Beyond Dieting

An organization committed to assisting, supporting and encouraging women and girls in their escape from the dieting trap. It offers on-going group support, workshops and seminars, as well as training for professionals about the health hazards of dieting. Its directors are Kim Chamberlain and Karena Shannon.

14/16 Proportion Plus

Aims to encourage designers and manufacturers to produce attractive, affordable clothes so that females in the 14/16+ size ranges have real choice of clothing.

You and the anti-diet movement

If avoiding fatness . . . is the main preoccupation of our lives, then what are we living for?

Roberta P. Seid

As you can see, there is plenty going on around the world, and this is not all. There will be other people and organizations out there that I don't know about.

Say 'no' to negative isolation and find something positive that will suit and help you. Read a book, attend a workshop or course, go to see the Fat Lip Readers' Theater, join Diet Breakers, invite a speaker to your women's group or organization, or buy the *Fat Chance* video.

Being involved in the anti-diet movement (at any level) can be a rewarding and enriching experience for you and provides us with the motivation to carry on working for a better way of living for all – which is what everyone deserves.

- Do you think you could benefit from discussing some of the issues raised in this book with other women?
- Are you keen to defeat the tyranny of thinness so that you and other women can get on with your lives without this unnecessary diversion?

I believe we are worth the effort and capable of turning things round to be more woman-friendly and more life- and soul-enhancing. Indeed, the fightback has already begun. Every day we get letters from women wanting more information about Diet Breakers, and at least once a week a student will contact me. She may be studying some aspect of the issue and want information, or she may ask to come and interview me. Sometimes students send us their work.

Recently Maria Louise Hill sent me her university project, which studies the effects of diet articles on women's body satisfaction. Maria's findings back up the DB questionnaires and the impact on us of the media and advertising. Her results suggest that women with eating disturbances are adversely affected by diet articles, and have greater body dissastisfaction after seeing such articles. Her study also suggests a high level of dieting behaviour in female undergraduates.

Where possible, I try to set time aside to give interviews to students as I realize that the bulk of the work to overturn the negative effects of the tyranny of thinness rests with young women – the next generation. The thought of thousands of young women in universities and colleges up and down the country forming groups, discussing and planning how to heal themselves and working forward is both moving and exciting, and I feel my blood rush at the prospect of 200,000 women out on the streets on International No Diet Day – reclaiming what is ours.

As Roberta Seid says,

It would be a tragedy, after twenty-five years of the women's movement, if women did not rebel against this 'religion' that threatens to sabotage their hard-won victories . . . This is a religion appropriate only for a people whose ideals do not extend beyond their physical existence, and whose vision of the future and of the past is strangely empty. Surely [we] can produce a worthier creed.

Women Against Tyranny of Thinness

Have you got to the end of this book and want more? Do you feel frustrated that improvements are not moving fast enough? Why not start a Women Against Tyranny of Thinness self-help group?

The aims and objectives of your group would be for the members to decide, but there are several possibilities:

- Your group could be run along the lines of the consciousness-raising groups of the seventies, where women got together weekly (usually at one member's home) and raised their consciousness awareness by sharing experiences. You could raise your consciousness about bodyism and how it has affected you, your friends and family and society generally, and what you need to do to break free individually and collectively.
- You could form a study group and discuss this book and others chapter by chapter (see Further Reading).
- You could form a support group and work your way through some of the exercises mentioned in this and other self-help books, such as *Transforming Body Image* or *The Women's Comfort Book*.
- You could form an action group and arrange activities such as letter writing and demonstrations that will empower you and other group members and help to get the word across to more

women. You could invite me and other activists to come and talk to your group.

- You could form a theatre group. Theatre is a wonderful way of heightening self-awareness, developing confidence and reaching other women.

How to start a WATT support group

If you already belong to a women's group or organization, talk to your colleagues and ask them if they are interested in starting a Women Against Tyranny of Thinness (WATT) self-help group with you.

Go and talk to the staff in your local library. Tell them about Diet Breaking and say that you want to start a group. Ask them to put a card on their notice board. Many libraries welcome local groups who want to advertise meetings, and often let them meet there too.

If your local council has a women's committee or equality officer contact her to see if she can help in any way (she may even be interested for herself). Likewise, if your local council has a community worker in your area, seek her/him out to see how they can help you get started.

If you are a student or a member of a trade union, go and talk with the women's officer of the union to ask for help in publicizing the meeting and any other help she can give.

But what if none of these options applies to you? Perhaps you are already a member of an organization or group where women are involved. Make a point of talking to the women there about Diet Breaking and tell them you would like to start a group. Ask if they are interested.

You could try putting a card in your local bookshop, health shop, newsagent's window or even ask at your doctor's surgery or health centre. You could contact the editor of the women's page of your local newspaper and ask her to run a little story about you starting a group, or you could place an advertisement in the local paper. It could read something like this:

WOMEN: Are you fed up with dieting and the tyranny of thinness? Do you want to meet like-minded women and break free to improve your body-image and self-esteem and beat the tyranny?

A free local self help Women Against Tyranny of Thinness (WATT) group is starting soon. For more details, contact: (give your name and telephone number).

Decide on a date and venue for the first meeting. Women are busy, so allow two or three weeks between the appearance of the story/advertisement and the first meeting.

When women contact you for more details of the group, ask them to think about what they would like from the group. If they are not sure, you could run through some of the ideas listed here. The group can then discuss various ideas and work out a programme of topics or agendas for future meetings, and decide how often you are going to meet. I would suggest once a week.

A group of between four and twelve people is ideal, but if there are just two of you, don't be disheartened – you at least have a partner to work with, and maybe other women will join you in due course. If the group has more than twelve people there may not be enough time and space for everyone to talk.

The first meeting

- Introduce yourself as the person who has organized the meeting, and explain that you would like to develop a WATT group to give support to yourself and other women.
- Tell the group what time you expect this first meeting to end. I would suggest that meetings do not last longer than two hours. People's concentration wanders and we all get tired.
- To help people feel safe, ask the group to agree that everything discussed in the meeting stays within the group. It would spoil the whole spirit of your group to back-bite or gossip about group members.
- Suggest that each person shares some information about themselves and why they have come, for up to five minutes each. This will help the group to relax and to get a feel for each other. When everyone who wants to has spoken, go back to anyone who hasn't and invite them to talk now if they wish. Don't press people to speak if they are reluctant, and make it clear that everyone, whether outgoing or reserved, is welcome.

At this initial meeting your group can decide what form it wants to take. There is no reason why it has to be one particular sort of group. You could decide to have different topics each week, or perhaps even to break into sub-groups within the meeting and then come back towards the end of the evening to share your experiences.

I suggest you agree a set of group guidelines which include the following:

- Frequency of meetings
- Starting and finishing times – and stick to them
- Venue for the meetings – where there will be no disturbances
- Only one person to speak at a time
- It is OK to disagree
- No advice-giving
- Rotate the chair of the meetings
- Agree to stick to the topic, and save chatting for before and after the meetings
- To send apologies if anyone can't get to a meeting

It will probably take a couple of weeks for the group to feel comfortable. You will need to give yourselves time to develop trust and a sense of togetherness, so don't try to rush things.

Suggested topics for discussion

- Dieting as a political issue
- Overcoming the tyranny of thinness
- Bodyism – how it works and how it affects me
- What I like about myself
- Improving my body image
- Taking care of myself and my own needs
- Building coalitions with other women
- Handling anger – mine and others'
- Coping with hunger
- Mothers and daughters as dieters
- Practising assertiveness

This list is intended simply to give you some ideas to help get your group started, and there are lots more things you could go on to discuss. Being in a group with like-minded women can be an exciting opportunity for personal empowerment – from raising your awareness and self-esteem to developing your listening and group skills, to organizing and chairing meetings, to goal setting and confidence building. There are no limits to what a bunch of women can achieve.

Come on, let's do it.

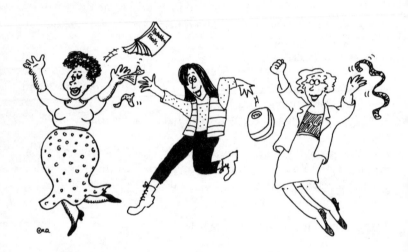

Useful Addresses

Advertising Standards Authority
Brook House
2–16 Torrington Place
London WC1E 7HN
Tel: 0171 580 5555

Alternative View
The Old Auction Mart
Station Approach
Godalming
GU7 1EU
United Kingdom
Tel: 0483 415225

AHELP
Eating Disorders Program
St Albans Psychiatric Hospital
Box 3608
Radford
VA 24143
USA
Tel: 800 3683468

Anorexia and Bulimia Nervosa Foundation of Victoria
1513 High Street
Glen Iris
Victoria 3146
Australia
Tel: 03 885 0318

ANRED (Anorexia Nervosa and Related Eating Disorders)
PO Box 5102
Eugene
Oregon 97405
USA
Tel: 503 344 1144

BBC
Head of Programme Complaints Unit
Broadcasting House
London W1A 1AA

BBC
Viewer and Listener Information
201 Wood Lane
London W12 7TS
Tel: 0181 743 8000

Beyond Dieting
PO Box 4452
Christchurch
New Zealand
Tel: 03 366 2248

Body Trust
2110 Overland Avenue
Suite 120
Billings
MT 59102
USA
Tel: 406 656 9417

Chicago Center for Overcoming Overeating
PO Box 48
Deerfield
IL 60015
USA
Tel: 708 853 1200

Council on Size and Weight Discrimination Inc.
PO Box 305
Mt Marion
NY 12456
USA
Tel: 914 679 1209

Diet Breakers
Barford St Michael
Banbury
OX15 OUA
United Kingdom
(Please always send a stamped addressed envelope)

Diet/Weight Liberation
Anabel Taylor Hall
Cornell University
Ithaca
NY 14853
USA
Tel: 607 257 0563

Eating Disorders Association
Sackville Place
44–48 Magdalen Street
Norwich
NR3 1JU
United Kingdom
Tel helpline: 01603 6214143 (9am–6.30pm, Monday–Friday)
Youth helpline (eighteen and under): 01603 765050 (4–6pm, Monday, Tuesday and Wednesday)

Fat Lip Readers' Theater
1148 Wilard Street
San Francisco
CA 94117
USA
Tel: 415 664 6842

Fat Women's Group
Wesley House
Wild Court
London WC2B 5AU
United Kingdom

Food Commission
Viking House
5–11 Worship Street
London EC2A 2BH
United Kingdom
Tel: 0171 628 7774

GUIDE (Guidance for Image, Dieting, and Eating)
University of Pennsylvania
Box 745 HUP
Philadelphia
PA 19104–4283
USA

Healthy Weight Journal
402 South 14th Street
Hettinger
ND 58639
USA
Tel: 701 567 2646

House of Commons
Westminster
London SW1

HUGS
Box 102A, RR#3
Portage La Prairie
Manitoba
Canada R1N 3A3
Tel: 204 254 1816

Independent Television Commission
33 Foley Street
London W1
Tel: 0171 255 3000

Institute of Trading Standards Administration
3–5 Hadleigh Business Centre
351 London Road
Hadleigh
Essex
SS7 2BT
United Kingdom
Tel: 0702 559922

Largesse
74 Woolsey Street
New Haven
CT 06513 3729
USA
Tel: 203 787 1624

Largely Positive
5531 N. Navajo Avenue
Glendale
WI 53217
USA
Tel: 414 454 6500
(Please always send a stamped addressed envelope)

NAAFA (National Association to Advance Fat Acceptance)
PO Box 188620
Sacramento
CA 95818
USA
Tel: 916 443 0303

National Center for Overcoming Overeating
315 W. 86th Street #17B
New York
NY 10024–3111
USA
Tel: 212 874 6596

National Education Office
Buskerud County
Torvhall
3017 Drammen
Norway
Tel: 32 896860
Fax: 32 895235

National Film Board of Canada
Customer Services D-10
PO Box 6100
Station Centre-ville
Montreal
Canada H3C 3H5

Norwegian Anorexia/Bulimia Association
Postboks 36
N-5001 Bergen
Norway
Tel: 55 326260
Fax: 55 325701

Office of Fair Trading
Field House
15–25 Breams Buildings
London EC4 1PR
Tel: 0171 242 2858

Press Complaints Commission
Salisbury Square
London EC4 8AE
Tel: 0171 353 1248

Pretty Big
1 The Dale
Wirksworth
Matlock
DE4 4EJ
United Kingdom
Tel: 0629 824949

14/16 Proportion Plus
Fashion and Interior Design College of New Zealand
PO Box 539
Westminster House
202 Cashel Street
Christchurch
New Zealand
Tel: 03 365 1578
Fax: 03 379 2310

Radiance
3839 Elston Avenue
Oakland
CA 94605
USA
Tel: 510 482 0680

Rump Parliament
PO Box 181716
Dallas
TX 75218
USA
Tel: 214 275 4449

Synergetic Workouts
PO Box 852
Maidenhead
SL6 1TP
United Kingdom
Tel: 0734 789 293

Transitions
24 Florence Street
Newtown
Wellington
New Zealand
Tel: 04 389 1076

Women at Large
12 Chancery Lane
Hawthorndene
SA 5051
Australia
Tel: 278 6499

Further Reading

Chapter 1

BOVEY, Shelley, *The Forbidden Body*, Pandora, 1994
DOLAN, Bridget and Inez Gitzinger (eds), *Why Women? Gender Issues and Eating Disorders*, Athlone Press, 1994
FALLON, Patricia, Melanie A. Katzman and Susan C. Wooley (eds), *Feminist Perspectives on Eating Disorder*, Guildford Press, 1994
WOLF, Naomi, *The Beauty Myth*, Vintage, 1992

Chapter 2

ASHWORTH, Sherry, *A Matter of Fat*, Signet, 1993
IND, Jo, *Fat Is a Spiritual Issue*, Mowbray, 1993

Chapter 3

BERG, Frances, *Health Risks of Obesity*, Healthy Weight Journal, 1992
BERG, Frances, *Health Risks of Weight Loss*, Healthy Weight Journal, 1992
OGDEN, Jane, *Fat Chance – The Myth of Dieting Explained*, Routledge, 1992
SANDERS, Tom and Peter Bazalgette, *You Don't Have to Diet*, Bantam, 1994

Chapter 4

LOUDEN, Jennifer, *The Woman's Comfort Book*, HarperCollins, 1992
PEDLER AND BOYDELL, *Managing Yourself*, Fontana, 1985
RODIN, Judith, *Body Traps*, William Morrow, 1992
SCHMIDT, Ulrike and Janet Treasure, *Getting Better Bit(e) by Bit(e)*, Lawrence Erlbaum Associates, 1994

Chapter 5

OMICHINSKI, Linda, *You Count, Calories Don't*, Tamos (Canada), 1992; Hodder & Stoughton (UK), 1996
The Journal of Gastronomy, Winter/Spring Issue 1993, The American Institute of Wine and Food

Chapter 6

LYONS, Pat and Debby Burgard, *Great Shape*, Bull Publishing, 1990
MAXWELL-HUDSON, Clare, *Complete Book of Massage*, Dorling Kindersley, 1994
MEICHENBAUM, Dr Donald, *Coping with Stress*, Century, 1993
MELPOMENE INSTITUTE FOR WOMEN'S HEALTH RESEARCH, *The Bodywise Woman*, Human Kinetics, 1993

Chapter 7

DAVIES, Philippa, *Your Total Image*, Piatkus, 1990
HUTCHINSON, Marcia Germaine, *Transforming Body Image – Learning to Love the Body You Have*, Crossing Press, 1985
MASON, Carla and Helen Villa Connor, *Timeless Beauty – Create Your Own Individual Style Whatever Your Size, Shape or Colouring*, Piatkus, 1994

Chapter 8

DICKSON, Anne, *A Woman in Your Own Right*, Quartet, 1982

Chapter 9

JOHNSON, Carol, *Largely Positive: Self Esteem Comes in All Sizes*, Doubleday, 1995

INDEX